SpringerBriefs in Public Health

SpringerBriefs in Public Health present concise summaries of cutting-edge research and practical applications from across the entire field of public health, with contributions from medicine, bioethics, health economics, public policy, biostatistics, and sociology.

The focus of the series is to highlight current topics in public health of interest to a global audience, including health care policy; social determinants of health; health issues in developing countries; new research methods; chronic and infectious disease epidemics; and innovative health interventions.

Featuring compact volumes of 55 to 125 pages, the series covers a range of content from professional to academic. Possible volumes in the series may consist of timely reports of state-of-the art analytical techniques, reports from the field, snapshots of hot and/or emerging topics, literature reviews, and in-depth case studies. Both solicited and unsolicited manuscripts are considered for publication in this series.

Briefs are published as part of Springer's eBook collection, with millions of users worldwide. In addition, Briefs are available for individual print and electronic purchase.

Briefs are characterized by fast, global electronic dissemination, standard publishing contracts, easy-to-use manuscript preparation and formatting guidelines, and expedited production schedules. We aim for publication 8–12 weeks after acceptance.

Emma R. Dorris • Liam Cleere • Thilo Kroll

Building the Ecosystem for Engaged Research

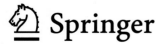 Springer

Emma R. Dorris
UCD Research
University College Dublin
Dublin, Dublin, Ireland

Liam Cleere
UCD Research
University College Dublin
Dublin, Dublin, Ireland

Thilo Kroll
UCD School of Nursing, Midwifery
and Health Systems
University College Dublin
Dublin, Dublin, Ireland

ISSN 2192-3698   ISSN 2192-3701   (electronic)
SpringerBriefs in Public Health
ISBN 978-3-031-82079-3   ISBN 978-3-031-82080-9   (eBook)
https://doi.org/10.1007/978-3-031-82080-9

This Springer imprint is published by the registered company Springer Nature Switzerland AG
The registered company address is: Gewerbestrasse 11, 6330 Cham, Switzerland

If disposing of this product, please recycle the paper.

This book is dedicated to the public contributors to research, in addition to the research, industry, public body and civil society administrators, managers and staff who are working to create a better research environment for all.

Preface

Research is changing. There is an increased focus on aligning strategic research with societal needs, expectations and values nationally and globally. Engaging the public and communities in different aspects of research design, conduct and dissemination can harness collective intelligence and improve the relationship between research and society. Opening research to societal voices can lead to more relevant outcomes and accelerate innovation. More open and inclusive approaches can reduce the distance between research and society, leading to greater impact for all stakeholders.

The authors of this book have a passion for research and have been striving to help researchers maximise the potential societal benefit from their research. Through these experiences, it has become increasingly clear that one of the greatest stumbling blocks that researchers face is the research ecosystem itself. The systems traditionally supporting research are based on old assumptions of who has a stake in research. These assumptions no longer hold true, yet the systems built upon are slow to adapt. In order to capitalise on the vast wealth of locally held knowledge for the benefit of research, fundamental changes in how we operate are required.

This book was written with research administrators, university leadership, policy professionals, research funders, community-based organisations, and non-governmental organisations in mind. It does not focus on project-level issues of engaged research, but rather on the organisational- and systems-level challenges and opportunities that exist. We present a critical reflection of engaged research as a systemic and dynamic process which continuously changes and which requires adaptation. The book does not lay out a firm road to achieve sustainable engaged research but can be considered as a map of the terrain with suggested pathways.

Dublin, Ireland

Emma R. Dorris
Liam Cleere
Thilo Kroll

Acknowledgements

The authors would like to thank and acknowledge Mark Coen, Katherine O'Donnell, Shane O'Donnell and Francesco Pilla for sharing their experiences and case studies with us. We would also like to thank David Bennett, who helped to curate and finesse the case studies.

About the Book

The heart of engaged research is the collaborative engagement with community stakeholders throughout the research cycle. The purpose is to improve the understanding of a phenomenon of public interest or concern together with, rather than for, members of the public. "Community" can refer to public or professional service and product users, policymakers, NGOs and the public at large.

Successfully embedding this into research culture requires buy-in from policy actors, research-performing organisations, academics and the public. This book discusses the ecosystem and infrastructure needed to successfully embed a culture of societally engaged research at a systems level. We discuss transformations required to achieve sustainable change and the actors responsible for implementing those transformations.

This brief book consists of four chapters. Chapter 1 provides an introduction and overview of the 'engaged research' concept and sets the scene. Chapter 2 discusses development of the engaged research ecosystem at the organisational level and the need for integrated approaches across units and services. Chapter 3 focuses on engaged research case studies, to demonstrate how engaged research can lead to greater research impact. Finally, Chapter 4 considers future trends in engaged research and how we can create adaptable environments for future challenges.

Contents

About the Authors

Emma R. Dorris, PhD, MPP, is the Engaged Research Manager in the Office of the Vice-President for Research, Innovation and Impact at University College Dublin in Ireland. She has a PhD in Molecular Medicine and a Master of Public Policy. She has direct experience in engaged research and in leading institutional reforms. Dr Dorris is currently managing the PPI Ignite Network at UCD, a core office of the national network aimed at innovating public and patient involvement in health and social care research. She also manages the development of centralised supports and infrastructure for engaged research across all disciplines in the university. Dr Dorris has an internationally recognised specialty in the involvement of public stakeholders in research that is not public facing. She is a member of the European Commission's community of practice on citizen engagement for knowledge valorisation and acts as an external advisor on a number of international funding and research improvement initiatives. She is a long-term advocate of open science practices and improved research culture.

Liam Cleere, MBA, is a Senior Manager in UCD Research and Innovation where he leads the Research Analytics and Impact team. The team helps to embed a culture of research engagement and impact in the university. He spearheaded the development and successful implementation of the research impact work programme at UCD. He has demonstrated thought leadership on the topic of impact and has presented to a range of audiences at both national and international conferences. Liam Cleere is the UCD representative on the Irish CoARA National Chapter and is involved in a number of national initiatives on the reform of research assessment. He has over 18 years of experience in research management. In addition, he has over 7 years of management consulting experience in Ireland and overseas. He has a degree in Mechanical Engineering and holds a Master of Business Administration (MBA).

Thilo Kroll, PhD, is a Full Professor of Health Systems Management at University College Dublin in Ireland. Over the past 30 years, he has conducted interdisciplinary research with a focus on disability-, rehabilitation- and health-related topics. Previously, he was the Co-Director of the interdisciplinary Social Dimensions of Health Institute (SDHI) of the Universities of Dundee and St Andrews in the UK. He closely collaborated with NGOs in the UK, USA, Norway, Germany and Ireland on projects focusing on disability, mental health, homelessness and violence. He advocates for systems and design thinking in research, education and practice. Currently, he is leading the implementation of public and patient involvement (PPI) in health- and social care-related work at UCD as part of the Irish HRB-funded National PPI Network.

List of Abbreviations

ABCD	Asset-Based Community Development
AID	Automated Insulin Delivery
ARC	Australian Research Council
CBPR	Community-Based Participatory Research
CDC	Centers for Disease Control and Prevention
DML	Donnybrook Magdalene Laundry
EDI	Equality, Diversity and Inclusion
ERA	European Research Area
GACER	Global Alliance on Community-Engaged Research
HE-BCI	Higher Education Business and Community Interaction
HEI	Higher Education Institutions
IP	Intellectual Property
IRB	Institutional Review Boards
KEF	Knowledge Exchange Framework
KTP	Knowledge Transfer Partnership
NCCPE	National Co-ordinating Centre for Public Engagement
NGO	Non-governmental organisations
NIH	National Institutes of Health
NIHR	National Institutes of Health Research
NIMHD	National Institute on Minority Health and Health Disparities
NMI	National Museum of Ireland
NSF	National Science Foundation
OECD	Organisation for Economic Co-operation and Development
OSTP	Office of Science and Technology Policy
PAR	Participatory Action Research
PCS	Passive Control Systems
PRC	Prevention Research Centers
R&I	Research and Innovation
REC	Research Ethics Committees
REF	Research Excellence Framework
RPO	Research Performing Organisation

RRI	Responsible Research and Innovation
S4P	Science for Policy
SDG	Sustainable Development Goal
SFI	Science Foundation Ireland
UCD	University College Dublin
UKRI	United Kingdom Research and Innovation
UN	United Nations
WHO	World Health Organization

List of Figures

List of Tables

Chapter 1
Introduction to Engaged Research

1.1 Introduction

The COVID-19 pandemic has generated considerable unease in the public regarding science (Kosyk et al. 2023; Hurst 2023). Scientists and healthcare experts, politicians, and legislators provided updates on the latest research findings, morbidity and mortality numbers, infection risk factors, and guidance on what the public could do to protect themselves and each other. Some information or public health measures needed to be more consistent, over or understated, and less confusing. Resentment and disillusionment with the scientific and political "establishment" have gained momentum over time. "Alternative facts" produced without rigorous science and often supported by self-styled experts took hold and were disseminated widely using "alternative" (social) media channels. In the aftermath of the pandemic, we now see widespread distrust of political institutions and alienation from evidence-based sciences. Governments, independent bodies, and scientists are reviewing what happened during the pandemic, trying to understand which decisions were correct at the time, what worked, and where measures taken were disproportionate or wrong. How did we get here? Essentially, as is now clear, what planted the roots of public distrust was the poor communication of actors in power and a lack of appropriate and ongoing direct engagement with public stakeholders. The pandemic may only be one area of societal relevance that illustrates how the approach to communication and engagement must change in global societies that are increasingly connected via social media platforms but may be locally disenfranchised or disengaged. Effective public engagement also refers to awareness of those who are not heard or visible. It requires targeted approaches to engagement that are timely, consistent, appropriate, and value the contributions and assets of the public stakeholders of all communities. People must feel listened to, respected, and seen as having the agency to actively shape research, practice, and policy.

E. R. Dorris et al., *Building the Ecosystem for Engaged Research*,
SpringerBriefs in Public Health, https://doi.org/10.1007/978-3-031-82080-9_1

This book attempts to characterise what is needed to design an ecosystem for engaged research with stakeholders in higher education. We suggest that we have only some of the answers. In addition, we will be unable to address all relevant issues in great depth and will refer the reader to additional reading materials. We consider the ecosystem of engaged research as a dynamic, constantly evolving place of openness and learning on how to work with public stakeholders to solve complex societal problems, such as pandemics. The authors strongly believe that engaged research will improve science, be more impactful, and produce better learning and guidance for all decision makers.

1.2   Foundations of Engaged Research

Since the first universities were founded, higher education has been considered a privileged place of study, discovery, and learning, mostly detached from the public but often funded through taxation. Academic freedom is a cherished principle. However, this freedom also meant that science's skills, power, and governance were in the hands of the elite, with often little accountability to the public.

We can trace the evolution of engaged research over the past 200 years. The origins and historical foundations of engaged university research can be traced back to the nineteenth century, often called community-engaged or public scholarship. In the United States, land-grant universities have been established to promote agricultural science and engineering education in response to the Industrial Revolution and evolving social needs. These institutions aim to serve the public by disseminating practical knowledge. The Morrill Act of 1862 facilitated the creation of these land-grant universities. Subsequently, the Smith-Lever Act of 1914 introduced cooperative extension services, extending university outreach to rural farmers and formalising university-public engagement in agricultural research.

In the mid-twentieth century, particularly after World War II, federal funding for research increased significantly in the United States, leading to university expansion. During this period, some universities played a notable role in advancing civil rights movements, with scholars and students collaborating with communities to address social issues. From the late twentieth century to the early twenty-first century, a renewed emphasis on public engagement expanded considerably; in the 1980s and the 1990s, community engagement advanced as critics highlighted universities' perceived detachment from society. This era saw the rise of service-learning programmes where students applied academic learning to community projects. The Carnegie Foundation for the Advancement of Teaching established initiatives, such as the Campus Compact in 1985, to promote community engagement. Consequently, engaged scholarship has emerged as a recognised field, fostering partnerships between universities and communities to co-produce knowledge.

In conjunction with historical developments in the United States, there has been a longstanding tradition of engaged research originating from the Global South. This tradition commenced during the colonial era when colonial powers established higher education institutions (HEIs). These institutions primarily served the interests of colonial administrations, training local elites to manage colonial affairs rather than addressing the broader needs of local communities.

In numerous countries in the Global South, a persistent endeavour has been to decolonise the education system. As part of this decolonisation process, universities emerged as centres for nationalist movements, seeking to redefine their roles to serve the needs of newly independent nations. During the 1960s and the 1970s, liberation and anti-colonial movements emphasised development and engaged research. Educators, such as Paulo Freire in Brazil, underscored the significance of education as a tool for liberation and the co-creation of knowledge with marginalised communities. In the 1970s and the 1980s, participatory action research (PAR) gained prominence in the Global South as a methodological approach involving community members as co-researchers. This approach has been widely adopted in Latin America, Africa, and Asia, empowering communities to identify and solve their problems. During the late 1980s and the 1990s, many countries underwent structural changes and introduced neoliberal reforms driven by international financial institutions. These policies often reduced funding for higher education and shifted towards market-oriented models. Indeed, the impact agenda is rooted in neoliberal ideology, focused on capturing academic research's return on public investment. As neoliberalism grew throughout the 1980s and 1990s, Western governments increasingly used market incentives for organisations to perform in the way that the government would like (Foucault et al. 2008). Early attempts at implementing the impact agenda were found to be too discipline specific, largely ignoring impact from the social and political sciences, and too focused on the concerns of business and industry (Donovan 2006). Research for societal benefit, without commercial application, was deprioritised. Despite these challenges, engaged research persisted frequently in collaboration with non-governmental organisations (NGOs) and grassroots movements. However, as political idealism evolved, so too did the definitions of research impact (Reed and Fazey 2021). Although there is no single definition, typically more modern definitions of non-academic impact emphasise the delivery of identifiable change or benefit outside the research community, be it political, social, cultural, or economic (Gunn and Mintrom 2016). This is closely aligned with the more recent acknowledgement of the value and growth of engaged research as an upstream driver of research impact.

In recent decades, engaged research has become more institutionalised in universities across the Global South through networks such as the Global Alliance on Community-Engaged Research (GACER) and the Talloires Network. Policy initiatives have also played a significant role, exemplified by South Africa's 1997 White Paper on Higher Education, which emphasised the role of higher education in community services and development. These approaches emphasise the importance of social justice and equity, interdisciplinarity and collaboration, cultural relevance, and indigenous knowledge.

1.3   Characterisation and Definition of Engaged Research

The concept of engaged research is multifaceted, with various definitions highlighting different aspects of this approach. Engaged research, which incorporates community-engaged or participatory research, represents a collaborative approach to conducting research that actively involves community members, stakeholders, or end users throughout the research process (Sanders Thomson et al. 2021). This approach has gained significant traction in recent years, reflecting a shift in how academia interacts with society.

A broad conceptual perspective is offered by the National Co-ordinating Centre for Public Engagement (NCCPE) in the United Kingdom, which describes engaged research as research that is undertaken with, for and by the public. This definition highlights the various ways the public can be involved in research, from being active participants to helping shape research questions and methodologies. The Australian National University adds an action-oriented dimension to its definition, describing engaged research as "the mutually beneficial interaction between researchers and external communities to share and generate knowledge to inform action". This definition emphasises the mutual benefit and the practical application of the knowledge generated.

The mutual benefit is also highlighted in the definition by Holliman and Warren (2017), which characterises engaged research as "research that is mutually beneficial to academic and non-academic participants and that contributes to both academic knowledge and societal impact". This definition underscores the reciprocal nature of engaged research in which researchers and community partners contribute to and benefit from the process.

The term public and patient involvement (PPI) has gained hold in health systems, services, and clinical research. The National Institutes of Health Research (NIHR) defines "Research being carried out 'with' or 'by' members of the public rather than 'to', 'about' or 'for' them. This includes, for example, working with research funders to prioritise research, offering advice as members of a project steering group, or carrying out part of the research".

In the United States, the Patient-Centred Outcome Research Institute (PCORI) defines it as "The meaningful involvement of patients, caregivers, clinicians, and other healthcare stakeholders throughout the entire research process". PPI typically entails active partnerships between researchers and the public or patients, characterised by collaboration in which individuals contribute to the research process and engage in shared decision-making. This involvement may span various research stages, including priority setting, design, implementation, dissemination of findings, and use evaluation. PPI contributors may serve on advisory committees, act as consultants and co-researchers, or assist in outreach efforts with community stakeholders. Generally, PPI enhances the relevance and quality of research by incorporating diverse perspectives, addressing real needs and concerns, and improving transparency and accountability. However, challenges persist in addressing power imbalances and achieving meaningful involvement and mutual benefit.

The connection between academic and community settings is emphasised in community-campus partnerships for health. In their definition, the dual goals of academic contribution and community well-being are explicitly stated. One such example is given by Virginia Commonwealth University, describing it as "a collaborative process between the researcher and community partner that creates and disseminates knowledge and creative expression to contribute to the discipline and strengthen the well-being of the community".

Instead of providing a single definition, Beaulieu et al. (2018) proposed a framework for understanding engaged research. Their framework identified three key dimensions: the extent of collaboration (from consultation to co-creation), the diversity of stakeholders involved, and the stages of the research process where engagement occurs. This framework allows for a more nuanced understanding of various forms and levels of engagement in research. University College Dublin (UCD) in Ireland has also presented an adapted framework based on the Wellcome Trust characterisation of public engagement. The "Avocado Public Engagement Spectrum" spans different layers, ranging from the outer edges of information sharing with the public to the innermost core of dialogue, shared decision-making, and partnership working with the public. The nature and degree of joint work between academic and public stakeholders involves collaboration, consultation, and informing/inspiring (UCD, 2018). The framework was developed with input from academic and public stakeholders.

Engaged research, as also reflected in the "Avocado framework", is not a single methodology but an approach involving various disciplines and a suite of research methods. The specific form can vary depending on the context, research questions, and stakeholders involved. This flexibility is both a strength and challenge for engaged research, allowing it to be adapted to different contexts.

It allows for bespoke use and implementation across different disciplines and contexts. However, it also necessitates clear communication and a shared understanding among stakeholders.

1.4   Importance and Societal Benefits of Engaged Research

Engaged research as an approach is timely and appropriate for research in the twenty-first century that seeks answers to complex societal challenges through interdisciplinary expertise and collaboration and a profound grounding in public stakeholder experiences and knowledge. Engaged research is particularly well-suited to addressing complex societal challenges. Many of today's "wicked" or complex problems (Brown et al. 2010), such as climate change, health inequalities, and social justice, require interdisciplinary approaches and diverse perspectives. Engaged research that incorporates public perspectives as well as multidisciplinary expertise has the potential to produce relevant, impactful, and ethically sound research outcomes.

Through the involvement of community stakeholders throughout the research process, engaged research ensures that the questions being asked, methods of study chosen, and solutions being developed are directly relevant to real-world problems. Greenhalgh et al. (2016) demonstrated that engaged research in health care led to more contextually appropriate interventions and improved implementation of research findings. Engaged research helps researchers anticipate barriers and enablers to interventions and services if they work closely with clinicians and patients as key stakeholders. This holds for the field of implementation science and knowledge translation. Bowen and Graham (2013) suggest that integrated knowledge translation approaches involving stakeholders throughout the research process can lead to better uptake of research findings. Participatory research methods can also significantly improve the research quality (Lindhult 2019). Jagosh et al. (2012) conducted a realist review of participatory research partnerships. They found that community knowledge and perspectives often led to more culturally appropriate research designs and more valid interpretations of data. The outreach and recruitment strategies and methodologies may be more relevant and acceptable when stakeholders are invited to share their views on appropriateness and acceptability.

Engaged research also plays a crucial role in empowering communities and building their capacity to address local issues (Brown & Stalker 2020; Sofolahan-Oladeinde et al. 2015). Wallerstein and Duran (2010) argue that community-based participatory research (CBPR) can help address health disparities by building community capacity and promoting social justice. This empowerment aspect is a crucial societal benefit of the engaged research approaches. Not all involved research approaches may change communities, but the experience of personal expertise, biographies, and local knowledge can empower stakeholders. This is particularly noteworthy in an era in which public trust in institutions, including universities, has declined. Stein et al. (2017) refer to the need to build trust. The growing public distrust in science and academia has dramatically boosted during the recent COVID-19 pandemic. Engaging research can help ensure it is conducted ethically, respecting the rights and interests of the communities involved. This is particularly crucial in research involving marginalised or vulnerable populations, as highlighted by Banks et al. (2013). Distrust in science may be substantial in communities that have been victims of unethical and inhuman practices in the name of science in the past.

In conclusion, engaged research offers a multifaceted approach to address many of the limitations of traditional research methodologies. Engaging research can significantly increase the societal benefits of academic research by enhancing relevance, improving quality, empowering communities, building trust, facilitating knowledge translation, addressing complex problems, and ensuring ethical practices.

1.5   Root Influences of Engaged Research

As we understand and practice today, engaged research has evolved from a rich tapestry of academic traditions and social movements. These diverse roots have contributed to their multifaceted nature and broad applicability in various fields.

One of the earliest influences on engaged research was action research, developed by psychologist Kurt Lewin in the 1940s. Action research emphasises the importance of conducting research in real-world settings, not just laboratories or highly controlled experiments. It is a problem-solving approach that has since underpinned a range of collaborative, change-oriented research methodologies. Building on this foundation, participatory action research (PAR) emerged in the 1970s. It was also heavily influenced by Paulo Freire's work on critical pedagogy, which has become prominent in Brazil. Based on the study by Baum et al. (2006), PAR emphasises the involvement of community members as co-researchers to empower marginalised groups through the research process itself. In this approach, community stakeholders can perceive themselves as part of the solution and not only as those associated with the problem.

Community-based participatory research (CBPR) was developed in the Health and Social Sciences as a specific approach to address health disparities. In particular, the work of Minkler and Wallerstein in the late 1990s and the early 2000s has been formative. Israel et al. (1998) describe how CBPR focuses on building equitable partnerships between researchers and communities, emphasising capacity building and long-term commitment to community well-being. For example, Indigenous Research Methodologies have profoundly impacted engaged research practices. Smith (2021) described how these approaches emphasise respect for indigenous knowledge and ways of knowing, further enriching the engaged research paradigm. These diverse influences have collectively shaped engaged research into the rich and multifaceted approach we see today.

1.6   Global Understandings and Practices of Engaged Research

CBPR has been widely adopted in North America, particularly in the United States and Canada. As Wallerstein et al. (2017) noted, this approach is especially prominent in public health and environmental studies, with a strong focus on addressing health disparities and social justice issues. The European context has witnessed the development of the "Responsible Research and Innovation" (RRI) framework. Owen et al. (2012) explain that this approach, which includes public engagement as a key pillar, aims to align research and innovation with societal values and needs, reflecting a broader European emphasis on social responsibility in science.

Australia and New Zealand have developed solid traditions for engaged research, particularly in their work with indigenous communities. Kukutai and Taylor (2016) highlight the emergence of "Indigenous Data Sovereignty" as a crucial principle in these contexts, reflecting a growing recognition of Indigenous rights and knowledge systems. Participatory Action Research has deep historical roots in Latin America and is heavily influenced by Paulo Freire's work. Fals-Borda and Rahman (1991) described how this approach emphasises social transformation and the empowerment of marginalised communities, reflecting the region's history of social movements and critical pedagogy. African-engaged research often focuses on developmental issues and decolonising research methodologies. Chilisa (2011) discusses the growing emphasis on "Ubuntu" research principles, prioritising communal relationships and mutual caring, reflecting African philosophical traditions. Engaged research has taken various forms in Asia. Hall and Tandon (2017) note that the Gandhian principles of self-reliance and community development have influenced countries such as India. East Asia has an increasing emphasis on university-industry collaboration in engaged research, reflecting different economic and development priorities.

Santos (2018) describes a growing movement to "decolonise" research methodologies across the Global South. This approach emphasises local and indigenous knowledge systems and challenges Western-centric research paradigms, reflecting a broader push for epistemic justice and diversity in knowledge production. These diverse global practices underscore the importance of cultural context in shaping engaged research approaches. They also highlighted the need for flexibility and cultural sensitivity when implementing engaged research principles across different settings, ensuring that the research reflects and responds to local needs, values, and ways of knowing.

Engaged research has gained global recognition, but its understanding and implementation vary significantly across regions and cultural contexts, reflecting diverse historical, social, and academic traditions. However, the core principles and values underpinning diverse approaches enable communication and collaboration worldwide.

1.7   Drivers of Engaged Research: Why Now?

The landscape of academic research has undergone significant changes in recent years, with engaged research gaining prominence owing to several interconnected factors. This shift reflects a broader transformation of how research is conceived, conducted, and valued in society. One of the primary drivers of this change is that funding bodies and policymakers now emphasise the societal impact of research, pushing academics to demonstrate greater accountability for how their work contributes to real-world changes. As Watermeyer (2014) noted, this focus on impact has led to a re-evaluation of research practices.

As mentioned, there has also been a growing distrust in expertise and institutions. This is particularly evident during the COVID-19 pandemic. In response to this challenge, engaged research offers a way to rebuild trust and credibility by increasing transparency and collaboration. Mazzucato (2018) argued that this approach can help bridge the gap between experts and the public, fostering a more inclusive and trustworthy research process. There has also been recognition that many contemporary societal challenges are complex and require a different approach to finding solutions. Climate change, social inequality, and public health crises require interdisciplinary approaches and diverse perspectives. Brown et al. (2010) highlighted how engaged research can provide the necessary framework for tackling these "wicked problems" by bringing together various stakeholders and forms of knowledge.

Technological advancements have facilitated research growth. With the rise of the Internet, communication and collaboration patterns and opportunities have changed. Knowledge sharing is not only the privilege of a few but has turned into a mass phenomenon. This has also led to valuing personal experiences and locally held knowledge alongside research evidence. As Bonney et al. (2014) point out, digital technologies have also made it easier to involve diverse stakeholders in research processes, opening up new possibilities for collaboration and participation. This has led to innovative forms of engaged research, such as citizen science projects and online participatory platforms. The emphasis on knowledge co-production has further propelled the growth of engaged research. Norström et al. (2020) argued that integrating different forms of knowledge—academic, practitioner, and community—is crucial for addressing complex problems. This approach recognises the value of diverse perspectives and experiences for generating meaningful and applicable research outcomes.

Ethical considerations have also significantly influenced the shift towards engaged research. There is growing recognition of the ethical imperative to involve communities in research that affects them, particularly in health and social research. Banks et al. (2013) emphasise the importance of addressing ethical challenges in community-based participatory research, highlighting the need for more inclusive and equitable research practices.

Finally, the push for open science and dissemination aligns well with the engaged research principles. Vicente-Saez and Martinez-Fuentes (2018) highlight how the open science movement, emphasising transparency and accessibility, complements the goals of engaged research.

These drivers have collectively created an environment where engaged research is more feasible and increasingly seen as necessary for addressing societal challenges and maintaining the relevance of academic research. As the research landscape continues to evolve, engaged research is likely to play an increasingly important role in shaping the creation, sharing, and application of knowledge.

1.8   The Current Policy Landscape

The policy landscape for engaged research has significantly transformed in recent years, reflecting a global shift towards more collaborative, impactful, and socially relevant research practices. This evolution is evident in the various initiatives and frameworks that have emerged across national and international contexts. The introduction of the Research Excellence Framework (REF) in 2014 marked a significant milestone in the United Kingdom. The REF incorporated "impact" as a critical component of research assessment, incentivising universities to engage more actively with non-academic partners and demonstrate the societal benefits of their research. As Watermeyer and Chubb (2019) notes, this has led to a new form of "competitive accountability" in academic life, where researchers are increasingly judged not only on their scholarly output but also on their ability to create tangible societal impact. At the European level, the Horizon Europe funding programme for 2021–2027 has further emphasised the importance of engaged research. The European Commission (2021) has structured this programme around "missions" designed to address significant societal challenges, encouraging collaborative and engaged approaches to research. This mission-oriented approach reflects a growing recognition of the need for research to address pressing social and environmental issues directly. The National Science Foundation (NSF) has incorporated the Broader Impacts criteria into its grant review process in the United States. Holbrook (2017) argued that this move encourages researchers to consider the societal implications of their work. However, he also cautioned that the future of the impact agenda depends on a careful revaluation of academic freedom. Australia has also embraced this trend, with the Australian Research Council (ARC) introducing an "Engagement and Impact Assessment" alongside its Excellence in Research for Australia framework. ARC's 2019 report highlights the growing importance of research engagement and its impact on society beyond academia.

On a global scale, the Global Research Council, a virtual organisation of science and engineering funding agencies worldwide, has emphasised the importance of public engagement in science. Their 2020 report on Responsible Research Assessment underscores the need for a more holistic approach to evaluating research that includes engagement and impact. The United Nations' Sustainable Development Goals (SDGs) have become critical drivers of engaged research. Nilsson et al. (2016) argue that the SDGs provide a crucial framework for aligning research with societal needs, encouraging more engaged and impactful research approaches across various disciplines.

Finally, the rise of Open Science policies in many countries and institutions has further supported the trend towards engaged research. The Organisation for Economic Co-operation and Development (OECD 2015) report on Making Open Science a Reality highlights how these policies often include public engagement and participatory research elements, further breaking down the barriers between academia and society.

These policy developments collectively reflect a broader shift in how research is valued and incentivised. They signal a move from traditional output-focused metrics towards a more holistic view of research that emphasises engagement, impact, and societal relevance. As this policy landscape continues to evolve, it will likely shape the practices and priorities of researchers and institutions further, driving the continued growth and development of engaged research approaches.

1.9 Engaged Research in Higher Education

Engaged research has become increasingly prominent in higher education institutions (HEIs) worldwide, fundamentally reshaping how universities approach their research missions. This shift reflects a broader transformation of the role of universities in society, moving towards more collaborative and socially responsive practices. One of the most significant changes occurred in institutional strategies and missions. As Trencher et al. (2014b) noted, many universities are now incorporating community engagement as a "third mission" alongside teaching and research. This new focus emphasises the university's role in addressing societal challenges and positioning HEIs as active contributors to social and environmental solutions. Specifically, universities have begun to emphasise public services and social responsibility as core elements of their missions. This commitment involves addressing societal challenges, promoting social justice, and improving the quality of life in local, national, and global communities. As part of this effort, many universities form partnerships with local communities, businesses, non-profit organisations, and local government agencies to achieve goals of mutual interest and foster social and economic development and service learning. Universities often play a significant role in the economic development of their region. This could include supporting local businesses, fostering innovation and entrepreneurship, and creating job opportunities through university-affiliated enterprises.

Most universities now have specific community outreach programmes and scholarships that target underserved and minority populations. Students and staff members are encouraged to engage in civic activities such as volunteering, which is intended to foster a culture of civic responsibility and shared leadership.

The United Nations SDGs have focused the attention of many HEIs on complex societal and real-world challenges. This has boosted community engagement, applied partnership research, and solution-oriented design practices. EU funding, for example, systematically encourages close collaboration between academic and non-academic industries and NGOs as well as professional partners to conduct research that leads to practical solutions for local issues, such as public health, environmental sustainability, and urban development. Universities and other HEIs contribute to their communities' cultural and artistic lives through public lectures, performances, exhibitions, and other events. These activities help enrich the community and provide educational and cultural benefits beyond campus. Universities implemented structural changes to support this shift. Sandmann and Watkins (2017) describe how some institutions have established dedicated offices or centres for community and scholarship engagement. These structures provide crucial support, resources, and coordination for engaged research initiatives, helping institutionalise these practices within the university system.

Another significant development is the integration of engaged research into the curricula. Fitzgerald et al. (2016) highlight how universities incorporate engaged research into undergraduate and graduate programmes, providing students with hands-on experience in collaborative, community-based study. This approach enriches students' learning experiences and helps cultivate a new generation of engaged scholars. Developing engaged research and PPI education modules at several universities has generated greater awareness and improved practical skills among researchers in various disciplines.

The interdisciplinary nature of engaged research drives new forms of collaboration among universities. One of the earlier models of interdisciplinary and intersectoral cooperation with continuing relevance was the triple helix model developed by Etzkowitz and Leydesdorff (1995) and Etzkowitz and Zhou (2017). It emphasises the importance of university-industry-government relationships in innovation, shaping ideas about engaged research in economic and regional development contexts. Since its first inception, latest iterations of the innovation model have been extended to quadruple and quintuple helices. The quadruple helix model expands the traditional triple helix framework (university, industry, government) by adding civil society and media to ensure innovation aligns with societal needs. It emphasises the public's role in shaping emerging technologies and the importance of media in influencing political and social realities. The quintuple helix model further integrates the environment with knowledge and innovation, focusing on sustainability and societal impact. This model is applied in areas like environmental change, democracy, and international cooperation. The five key subsystems (helices) are (1) education system: creates human capital (students, researchers); (2) economic system: focuses on economic capital (entrepreneurship, money); (3) natural environment: provides natural capital (resources, biodiversity); (4) media and culture: combines social and information capital (traditions, media), and (5) political system: organises laws, policies, and political capital. These helices work together to drive innovation and sustainable development.

Universities have forged new partnerships and networks to facilitate research. Watson et al. (2011) describe how institutions form long-term collaborations with community organisations, government agencies, and industry partners. The Talloires Network connects universities globally through civic engagement, fostering international cooperation and knowledge sharing (Hollister et al. 2012).

As engaged research has become more prevalent, HEIs are developing new evaluation and impact assessment methods. Furco (2010) discusses how universities move beyond traditional academic measures to establish metrics that capture the broader societal impact of engaged research. This shift reflects a growing recognition of the need to demonstrate engaged scholarship's value to academic and non-academic stakeholders. At UCD, for example, engaged research contributions are recognised within the career development framework and are routinely entered into a centrally held database.

Finally, many universities are expanding their research initiatives. Larsen (2016) examines how institutions address international development challenges and foster global citizenship through engaged research practices. This global engagement broadens university research's scope and impact while raising essential questions about cross-cultural collaboration and ethical engagement. These developments collectively reflect a broader shift in how universities conceptualise their societal roles. This book reviews some of the challenges and solutions to fully institutionalising engaged research within traditional academic structures and cultures.

1.10 The Need for a New Ecosystem of Engaged Research

1.10.1 Reimagining Research: Engaged Approaches and Power Dynamics

Traditional research approaches in higher education institutions (HEIs) often suffer from a disconnect between academic priorities and public needs, leading to limited practical applicability and a "knowledge-to-action gap" (Graham et al. 2006). These models are typically researcher driven, with minimal input from communities affected by the research (Stilgoe et al. 2014). The disconnect results in academic knowledge that, while theoretically robust, may need more relevance in addressing real-world challenges (Van de Ven and Johnson 2006).

Additionally, traditional approaches often exclude diverse perspectives, particularly those of marginalised groups such as individuals with learning disabilities or low literacy skills (Kroll et al. 2014; Jahagirdar et al. 2012; Browne and Dorris 2022). This exclusion can lead to biased findings, reinforce social inequalities, and limit the comprehensiveness of research outcomes (Jagosh et al. 2012). Moreover, ethical concerns surrounding research on vulnerable populations are significant, with a lack of community stakeholder engagement potentially leading to exploitative practices (Banks et al. 2013). Another critical issue is the need for more dissemination of research findings across academic circles. Academic publications, the primary output of traditional research, often must be made available to non-academic audiences, confining valuable knowledge to academia (Watermeyer 2014).

1.10.2 The Shift Towards Engaged Research and New Power Dynamics

There has been a growing movement towards more engaged, participatory, and socially responsive research models in response to these shortcomings. Engaged research seeks to bridge the gap between academia and society, ensuring that research is rigorous but also relevant, accessible, and beneficial to the broader public. This shift fundamentally alters power dynamics in the research process, challenges traditional hierarchies, and fosters equitable relationships between researchers and communities (Minkler 2004). A vital aspect of this shift is the reframing of community members as active partners in the research process rather than passive subjects. CBPR, for example, views community members as co-creators of knowledge, thus enhancing the relevance and applicability of research (Israel et al. 1998). Shared decision-making is another cornerstone of engaged research. In CBPR, decisions about research questions, methodologies, and dissemination strategies are made collaboratively with community partners, ensuring that the research serves community needs (Wallerstein and Duran 2010). This approach also emphasises capacity building within communities, empowering them to conduct enquiries and enhancing their ability to address future challenges (Minkler and Wallerstein 2008). CBPR explicitly seeks to mitigate power imbalances, fostering more equitable research practices and outcomes that serve community needs better (Freudenberg and Tsui 2014). Additionally, engaged research emphasises reciprocal learning, in which researchers and community members benefit from mutual exchanges of knowledge, building trust, and long-term partnerships (Maiter et al. 2008).

Engaged research also democratises knowledge by acknowledging the value of diverse knowledge systems, including local and indigenous knowledge, thus challenging the traditional primacy of academic expertise (Hall and Tandon 2017). This movement is part of broader efforts to decolonise research and address historical knowledge production and validation imbalances. Academics involved in engaged research are encouraged to critically reflect on their power and privileges, actively working to share power with community partners, which leads to more ethical and effective research practices (Muhammad et al. 2015).

1.10.3   Value Shifts

Engaged research reflects a significant shift in how research is valued and conducted within academia, emphasising societal impact, inclusivity, and ethical
responsibility over traditional academic output. This transformation involves reimagining universities as active participants in societal problem-solving rather than
isolated "ivory towers" (Fitzgerald et al. 2016). The shift also includes a growing
focus on transdisciplinarity, which integrates diverse forms of knowledge to address
complex societal issues (Klein 2015). The increasing value placed on sustainability,
social responsibility, and equity underscores the broader societal demand for
research that addresses environmental and social challenges directly (Trencher et al.
2014a; Mertens 2007, 2021). Co-creation and collaboration with communities have
become central, reflecting the need for collective approaches to research that move
beyond the traditional single-researcher model (Gerke et al. 2023; Greenhalgh
et al. 2016).

Additionally, transparency and openness in research are increasingly valued,
aligning with the principles of open science (Vicente-Saez and Martinez-Fuentes
2018). Researchers are also encouraged to be reflexive, critically examining the
positionality and values embedded in their work and may use qualitative methods to
pursue introspection and open science (Humphreys et al. 2021; Finlay 2002).

How knowledge is valued in engaged research marks a departure from traditional
approaches by emphasising the value of community knowledge and assets in the
research process. This approach, rooted in the Asset-Based Community Development
(ABCD) model, recognises and leverages existing community strengths rather than
solely focusing on deficits (Martin-Kerry et al. 2023; Kretzmann and McKnight
1993). Engaged research also taps into tacit knowledge—unspoken, context-specific
insights held by community members—which can be invaluable in innovation and
problem-solving (Nonaka and Takeuchi 1995) as well as unique stakeholder assets or
capacities (Sáinz-Ruiz et al. 2021; Mueller et al. 2020; McPherson et al. 2020).
Incorporating local and indigenous knowledge into research is increasingly recognised as crucial for addressing complex societal challenges, particularly in sustainability science (Chilisa 2017). This inclusive approach values the contributions of
diverse knowledge systems and seeks to decolonise research practices. Co-production
of knowledge, where academic and community expertise are combined, is central to
this model, challenging traditional power dynamics and enhancing the relevance and
applicability of research (Ostrom 1996). Cultural competence is essential in this context, requiring researchers to respect diverse ways of knowing and navigating the ethical challenges of engaging with communities (Minkler 2004). Capacity building and
knowledge translation are critical components of knowledge valorisation. Engaged
research often leads to developing new skills and knowledge within communities,
empowering them to address issues independently (Wallerstein and Duran 2010).
Moreover, translating research findings into accessible and valuable forms ensures
that the knowledge produced benefits the communities involved (Graham et al. 2006).

Engaged research enhances academic work's societal impact and relevance and
fosters more equitable and sustainable approaches to addressing societal challenges.
This model empowers researchers and communities by recognising and valuing the

multidirectional flow of knowledge between academia and communities, contributing to a more inclusive and impactful research landscape.

1.11   Creating a New "Ecosystem" of Engaged Research

In the context of engaged research, the concept of an "ecosystem" represents a paradigm shift in how we understand and implement research partnerships. This holistic, interconnected approach borrows from ecological thinking to emphasise engaged research environments' complex, dynamic, and interdependent nature.

The core of this ecosystem approach is the recognition of the interconnectedness of its stakeholders, both within and between institutions. This perspective encourages researchers and stakeholders to consider the broader implications of their actions and decisions, recognising that changes in one part of the system can have far-reaching effects. How research is conducted depends on stakeholders' purposeful, dynamic interaction, which requires an agile infrastructure with appropriate support. The diverse stakeholder landscape may include researchers, academic institution members, community members, policymakers, funders, and practitioners. This multi-stakeholder approach ensures that research is informed by various perspectives and experiences, leading to more comprehensive and relevant outcomes.

Universities and research institutions are increasingly adopting learning organisation principles, as Senge (2006) described. This approach emphasises continuous learning and adaptation at the institutional level, enabling organisations to respond more to changing societal needs and research paradigms. Institutions must implement self-reflexive and adaptive processes at all levels to allow engaged research. University research ethics committees, finance departments, human resources, estate departments, and leadership at all levels must be agile and adapt their processes to meet the needs of diverse stakeholders, as discussed in Chap. 2. By adopting this ecosystem approach, researchers and stakeholders can better navigate the complexities of engaged research, fostering more resilient, adaptive, and impactful partnerships. However, it also presents challenges, requiring new ways of thinking about research organisation, funding, and evaluation. As engaged research continues to evolve, the ecosystem metaphor provides a valuable framework for understanding and nurturing the complex relationships underpinning effective community-academic partnerships.

1.11.1   Stakeholder Identification and Management in an Engaged Research Ecosystem

The ecosystem of engaged research involves diverse stakeholders, each of whom plays a crucial role in the research process. Understanding and effectively managing these stakeholders are essential for the success of research initiatives. HEIs are critical stakeholders at the core of this ecosystem, including administration and support staff, academic researchers, faculty members, postdoctoral researchers, and graduate students from various disciplines (Fitzgerald et al. 2016).

The term "community" denotes non-academic stakeholders and encompasses a diverse group of public entities, some with idealistic and others with commercial remits and interests, such as non-governmental organisations and businesses. Community organisations such as non-profit organisations and grassroots groups also play a significant role. Wallerstein and Duran (2010) highlight how these entities represent community interests and can serve as crucial bridges between academic researchers and local communities. Individual community members or "representatives" have different motivations to engage in shared projects with academic researchers. In some cases, there is a conflation of advocacy and engagement as co-researchers. The boundaries between advocacy and participatory research are blurred. However, this may be less so in other types of research. Similarly, for-profit partners or businesses may have different expectations than NGO partners working with HEIs. Academic and non-academic stakeholders must set out different expectations at the outset of any partnership.

Funders, including government agencies and private ones, are crucial stakeholders. They do not only provide financial research support but also define research priorities and approaches. Moreover, their emphasis on and openness toward engaged research is crucial to transforming the ecosystem of universities to work in partnership with communities. Policymakers at the local, regional, and national levels who influence the strategic funding investments for higher education and finding bodies are critical stakeholders. Cairney and Oliver (2017) discussed the complex relationship between research and policy, highlighting the potential for research findings to inform policy decisions. Non-governmental organisations (NGOs) often contribute valuable perspectives and resources. Brown et al. (2012) discussed how these organisations can help frame research engagement in ways that democratise knowledge production. Professional associations that represent specific fields are also important stakeholders. Greenhalgh et al. (2016) discuss how these groups can contribute to achieving research impact through co-creation in community-based settings. Finally, undergraduate and graduate students are key stakeholders. They are the next generation of researchers whose values and skills will drive how research is conducted.

Identifying these stakeholders is the first step. It is crucial to understand their interests, capacities, and potential contributions to the research process. Moreover, new stakeholders may emerge as research evolves, and existing relationships may change, requiring ongoing attention to stakeholder management throughout the research process. One of the most critical challenges in engaged research is stakeholder management. This involves understanding and balancing different perspectives, values, expectations, and contributions, which require a strategic and structured approach.

Roles, responsibilities, and boundaries must be negotiated and clearly articulated for each stakeholder at the outset of the collaboration. When stakeholders understand their specific tasks and expectations, it minimises confusion and ensures everyone is working towards the same goals. Existing resources are available to help with project-level expectation setting (Dorris et al. 2023; PARADIGM 2024). According to Jagosh et al. (2015), a realist evaluation of community-based participatory research highlights that well-defined roles enhance partnership synergy and build participant trust. Allowing for role adjustments as the project evolves and stakeholder capacities or interest changes is necessary for sustained engagement. Greenhalgh et al. (2016) advocate for achieving research impact through co-creation in community-based health services, which requires flexible roles to adapt to changing circumstances and emerging needs.

Power sharing may be particularly challenging for academic researchers who are used to setting the research agenda and implementing their research plan. Genuine, engaged research necessitates a process of relationship and trust building. This is facilitated by shared decision-making and by transparently assessing the value of community stakeholders' contributions. It should also be adequately remunerated.

Continuous, transparent, and inclusive communication ensures that all partners can effectively and meaningfully contribute to the process. A failure to step back from purely academically focused language can alienate partners and exacerbate power differences. Apart from choosing an appropriate language, information must be regularly and transparently shared.

It is crucial to provide training and support to enable all stakeholders to participate effectively in the research process. Community stakeholders may be trained in the requirements of research and related processes. In contrast, academic training may help them understand communities, choose appropriate approaches for engaging with stakeholders, and value their contributions. This also includes effective conflict resolution strategies, including mediation, open dialogue, and establishing a clear protocol for handling disputes for all stakeholders.

Acknowledging all stakeholder contributions to the research process is essential for the continued engagement and motivation of all partners. Different forms of acknowledgement and recognition may be necessary for various stakeholders. They may include authorship in critical publications, tangible, monetary rewards for the community partners, or visibility of the work to influence changes in policy and practice. In any case, what form of recognition is expected and feasible should be determined from the start.

One of the hallmarks of engaged research is relationship building. This is a process and is different from ad hoc relationships for short-term research projects. Therefore, developing strategies for sustaining stakeholder engagement over time is essential. Sustainability planning is critical to ensure that the research will have lasting impacts. Sustainability can be achieved through building long-term partnerships, securing ongoing funding, and embedding research into community structures.

Finally, reviewing and evaluating how well and what works in the engagement process is essential. Feedback mechanisms, reflective practices, and iterative adjustments help to maintain the relevance and effectiveness of engagement strategies (Khodyakov et al. 2013).

1.12 Summary and Key Messages

The landscape of academic research is undergoing a profound transformation, driven by the growing recognition that traditional research approaches often fail to address complex societal challenges and deliver meaningful impacts. This realisation has led to engaged research, a collaborative approach that seeks to bridge the gap between academia and society. Engaged research represents a paradigm shift from the conventional "ivory tower" model of knowledge production. It acknowledges that valuable expertise exists within academic institutions and communities, organisations, and diverse stakeholder groups. By fostering partnerships between researchers and those affected by or interested in research, engaged research aims to co-create rigorous and relevant knowledge.

However, the transition to this new research model is challenging. This requires a fundamental reimagining of the research ecosystem, one that can support and nurture these collaborative endeavours. This new ecosystem must be able to address several key issues. First, it must facilitate a shared understanding of engaged research among diverse stakeholders. This involves breaking down disciplinary silos, challenging traditional notions of expertise, and developing a common language that resonates across academic and non-academic contexts. Second, the new ecosystem must be adept at managing stakeholders' often conflicting values and expectations. It needs to balance the scholarly pursuit of knowledge with the practical needs of communities, the requirements of funders, and broader societal impact. Third, building trust and equitable relationships must be prioritised. This involves acknowledging and addressing power imbalances, ensuring genuine representation and inclusion, and valuing diverse forms of knowledge and contribution.

Furthermore, the new ecosystem must be agile, adaptive, and capable of responding to emerging needs and changing circumstances. This requires flexibility, often at odds with the traditional academic structures and processes. The ecosystem must also support the negotiation of expectations among stakeholders, ensuring that research benefits are equally distributed and that all parties find value in collaboration. Most importantly, this new ecosystem must foster a culture of mutual learning and shared benefits. The engaged research process is as valuable as its outcomes, with capacity building and relationship development being critical products of the research process.

The development of such an ecosystem is a prominent feature. This requires changes at multiple levels, from individual researchers and community partners to academic institutions, funding bodies, and policymakers. It calls for new skills, success metrics, reward structures, and ways of conceptualising and conducting research. The increasing complexity of societal challenges drives the need for this new ecosystem, the demand for more relevant and impactful research, and the ethical imperative of conducting research with and for communities rather than on them. It represents a shift towards a more democratic, inclusive, and socially responsive model of knowledge production.

In conclusion, while creating this new ecosystem of engaged research is challenging, it also has potential. It offers the promise of research that is more relevant, ethical, and impactful. As we move forward, embracing this new paradigm will be crucial for academia to maintain its relevance and fulfil its responsibility to society in the twenty-first century.

Key Messages
1. Engaged research has a long history and is grounded in various philosophical and political traditions globally.
2. Complex societal challenges necessitate innovative, agile, and interdisciplinary forms of research that engage non-academic stakeholders and the public genuinely and effectively.
3. Policymakers, universities, and funding bodies have begun to recognise the value and innovative potential of public engagement in research and seek to build capacity in this area.
4. Higher education institutions need to adapt and transform to facilitate engaged research processes, which require new forms of collaboration and trusting relationships in an agile support ecosystem.

References

Banks S, Armstrong A, Carter K, Graham H, Hayward P, Henry A, et al. Everyday ethics in community-based participatory research. Contemp Soc Sci. 2013;8:263–77.

Baum F, MacDougall C, Smith D. Participatory action research. J Epidemiol Community Health. 2006;60(10):854–7.

Beaulieu M, Breton M, Brousselle A. Conceptualizing 20 years of engaged scholarship: a scoping review. PLoS One. 2018;13(2):e0193201.

Bonney R, Shirk J, Phillips TB, Wiggins A, Ballard HL, Miller-Rushing AJ, et al. Next steps for citizen science. Science. 2014;343:1436–7.

Bowen SJ, Graham ID. From knowledge translation to engaged scholarship: promoting research relevance and utilization. Arch Phys Med Rehabil. 2013;94(1 Suppl):S3–8.

Brown M-E, Stalker KC. Consensus organizing and community-based participatory research to address social-structural disparities and promote health equity. Fam Community Health. 2020;43:213–20.

Brown V, Harris J, Russell J. Tackling wicked problems through the transdisciplinary imagination 2010.

Brown K, Keast R, Waterhouse J, Murphy G, Mandell M. Co-Management to Solve Homelessness: Wicked Solutions for Wicked Problems. In: Pestoff V, Brandsen T, Verschuere B, editors. New Public Governance, the Third Sector and Co-Production. 1 ed. New York: Routledge; 2012. p. 211–26.

Browne J, Dorris ER. What can we learn from a human-rights based approach to disability for public and patient involvement in research? Front Rehabil Sci. 2022;3:44.

Cairney P, Oliver K. Evidence-based policymaking is not like evidence-based medicine, so how far should you go to bridge the divide between evidence and policy? Health Res Policy Sys. 2017;15(1):35.

Chilisa B, (Ed.). Indigenous research methodologies 2011.

Chilisa B. Decolonising transdisciplinary research approaches: an African perspective for enhancing knowledge integration in sustainability science. Sustain Sci. 2017;12:813–27.

Donovan C. An instrument too blunt to judge sharp minds. Times Higher Education Supplement. 2006;11. ISSN 0049-3929

Dorris ED, Delaney S, Dunne N, Keegan D, Mulroy D, Murphy J. Expectations of engagement template document for PPI relationships. Figshare. 2023:24026442.v2.

Etzkowitz H, Leydesdorff L, editors. The triple helix – university-industry-government relations: a laboratory for knowledge based economic development. EASST Rev. 1995;14:14–9.

Etzkowitz H, Zhou C, editors. The triple helix: university–industry–government innovation and entrepreneurship. 2nd ed. Routledge; 2017.

European Commission. Communication from the Commission to the European Parliament, the Council, the European Economic and Social Committee and the Committee of the Regions on European Missions. Luxembourg: Publications Office of the European Union, 2021; 2021. https://doi.org/10.2777/084922

Fals-Borda O, Rahman MA. Action and knowledge: breaking the monopoly with participatory action research. New York: Apex; 1991.

Finlay L. Negotiating the swamp: the opportunity and challenge of reflexivity in research practice. Qualitative Research. 2002;2(2):209–30. https://doi.org/10.1177/146879410200200205

Fitzgerald HE, Bruns K, Sonka ST, Furco A, Swanson LE. The centrality of engagement in higher education: reflections and future directions. J High Educ Outreach Engagem. 2016;20:245–54.

Foucault M, Davidson AI, Burchell G. The birth of biopolitics: lectures at the Collège de France, 1978–1979. Springer; 2008.

Freudenberg N, Tsui E. Evidence, power, and policy change in community-based participatory research. Am J Public Health. 2014;104(1):11–4.

Furco A. The engaged campus: toward a comprehensive approach to public engagement. Br J Educ Stud. 2010;58:375–90.

Gerke D-M, Uude K, Kliewe T. Co-creation and societal impact: toward a generic framework for research impact assessment. Evaluation. 2023;29:489–508.

Graham ID, Logan J, Harrison MB, Straus SE, Tetroe J, Caswell W, et al. Lost in knowledge translation: Time for a map? Journal of Continuing Education in the Health Professions. 2006;26(1):13–24. https://doi.org/10.1002/chp.47

Greenhalgh T, Jackson C, Shaw S, Janamian T. Achieving research impact through co-creation in community-based health services: literature review and case study. Milbank Q. 2016;94(2):392–429.

Gunn A, Mintrom M. Higher Education Policy Change in Europe: Academic Research Funding and the Impact Agenda. European Education. 2016;48(4):241–57. https://doi.org/10.108 0/10564934.2016.1237703

Hall BL, Tandon R, editors. Decolonization of knowledge, epistemicide, participatory research and higher education. Res All. 2017;1(1):6–19.

Holbrook JB. The future of the impact agenda depends on the revaluation of academic freedom. Palgrave Commun. 2017;3(1):39.

Holliman, R. & Warren, C., (2017) "Supporting future scholars of engaged research", Research for All 1(1), 168–184. https://doi.org/10.18546/RFA.01.1.14

Hollister RM, Pollock JP, Gearan M, Reid J, Stroud SE, Babcock E. The Talloires network: a global Coalition of Engaged Universities. J High Educ Outreach Engagem. 2012;16:81–102.

Humphreys L, Lewis NA, Sender K, Won AS. Integrating qualitative methods and Open Science: five principles for more trustworthy research*. J Commun. 2021;71(5):855–74.

Hurst LD. Why some people don't trust science—and how to change their minds. In: The Conversation; 2023. https://theconversation.com/why-some-people-dont-trust-science-and-how-to-change-their-minds-219579.

Israel BA, Schulz AJ, Parker EA, Becker AB. Review of community-based research: assessing partnership approaches to improve public health. Annu Rev Public Health. 1998;19:173–202.

Jagosh J, Macaulay AC, Pluye P, Salsberg J, Bush PL, Henderson J, et al. Uncovering the benefits of participatory research: implications of a realist review for health research and practice. Milbank Q. 2012;90(2):311–46.

Jagosh J, Bush PL, Salsberg J, Macaulay AC, Greenhalgh T, Wong G, et al. A realist evaluation of community-based participatory research: partnership synergy, trust building and related ripple effects. BMC Public Health. 2015;15(1):725.

Jahagirdar D, Kroll T, Ritchie K, Wyke S. Using patient reported outcome measures in health services: A qualitative study on including people with low literacy skills and learning disabilities. BMC Health Services Research. 2012;12(1):431. https://doi.org/10.1186/1472-6963-12-431

Khodyakov D, Stockdale S, Jones A, Mango J, Jones F, Lizaola E. On measuring community participation in research. Health Educ Behav. 2013;40(3):346–54.

Klein JT. Reprint of "discourses of transdisciplinarity: looking back to the future" ☆. Futures. 2015;65:10–6.

Kosyk A, Kirsten A, Scheu AM, Uth B. COVID-19 sceptics' attitudes and expectations toward the media: understanding the role of moral judgements on trust and distrust in journalistic communication on COVID-19. Stud Commun Media. 2023;12:155.

Kretzmann JP, McKnight JL. Building communities from the inside out: a path toward finding and mobilizing a Community's assets. Institute for Policy Research, Northwestern University; 1993. Contract No.: Report

Kroll T, Wyke S, Jahagirdar D, Ritchie K. If patient-reported outcome measures are considered key health-care quality indicators, who is excluded from participation? Health Expectations. 2014;17(5):605–7. https://doi.org/10.1111/j.1369-7625.2012.00772.x

Kukutai T, Taylor J. In: Kukutai T, Taylor J, editors. Indigenous data sovereignty: toward an agenda. ANU Press; 2016.

Larsen K, Bandara DC, Esham M, Unantenne R. Promoting university-industry collaboration in Sri Lanka: status, case studies, and policy options. 1st ed. Washington, DC: World Bank Group; 2016.

Lindhult E. Scientific excellence in participatory and action research: part I. Rethinking Research Quality. Technol Innov Manag Rev. 2019;9(5):6–21.

Maiter S, Simich L, Jacobson N, Wise JB. Reciprocity. Action Res. 2008;6:305–25.

Martin-Kerry JM, McLean J, Hopkins T, Morgan A, Dunn L, Walton RT, et al. Characterizing asset-based studies in public health: development of a framework. Health Promot Int. 2023;38

Mazzucato M. The value of everything: makers and takers in the global economy. London: Allen Lane, an imprint of Penguin Books; 2018.

McPherson MQ, Friesner DL, Bozman CS. Mapping the interrelationships between community assets. Int J Soc Econ. 2020;47:1299.

Mertens DM. Transformative Paradigm:Mixed Methods and Social Justice. Journal of Mixed Methods Research. 2007;1(3):212–25. https://doi.org/10.1177/1558689807302811

Mertens DM. Transformative Research Methods to Increase Social Impact for Vulnerable Groups and Cultural Minorities. International Journal of Qualitative Methods. 2021;20:16094069211051563. https://doi.org/10.1177/16094069211051563

Minkler M. Ethical challenges for the "outside" researcher in community-based participatory research. Health Educ Behav. 2004;31(6):684–97.

Minkler M, Wallerstein N. Community-based participatory research for health: from process to outcomes. 2nd; 2. Aufl.; 2; ed. San Francisco, CA: Jossey-Bass; 2008.

Mueller D, Hoard S, Roemer KF, Sanders C, Rijkhoff SAM. Quantifying the community capitals framework: strategic application of the community assets and attributes model. Community Dev. 2020;51:535–55.

Muhammad M, Wallerstein N, Sussman AL, Avila M, Belone L, Duran BM. Reflections on researcher identity and power: the impact of positionality on community based participatory research (CBPR) processes and outcomes. Crit Sociol. 2015;41:1045–63.

Nilsson M, Griggs DJ, Visbeck M. Policy: map the interactions between sustainable development goals. Nature. 2016;534:320–2.

Nonaka I, Takeuchi H. The knowledge-creating company: how Japanese companies create the dynamics of innovation. New York/Oxford: Oxford University Press; 1995.

Norström AV, Cvitanovic C, Löf MF, West S, Wyborn C, Balvanera P, et al. Principles for knowledge co-production in sustainability research. Nat Sustainability. 2020;3:182–90.

OECD. Making open science a reality. OECD; 2015

Ostrom E. Crossing the great divide: coproduction, synergy, and development. World Dev. 1996;24(6):1073–87.

Owen R, Macnaghten P, Stilgoe J. Responsible research and innovation: from science in society to science for society, with society. In: Emerging technologies: ethics, law and governance; 2012.

PARADIGM. (2024) PE Toolbox.. Available from: https://imi-paradigm.eu/petoolbox/

Reed MS, Fazey I. Impact Culture: Transforming How Universities Tackle Twenty First Century Challenges. Frontiers in Sustainability. 2021;2. https://doi.org/10.3389/frsus.2021.662296

Sáinz-Ruiz PA, Sanz-Valero J, Gea-Caballero V, Melo P, Nguyen TH, Suárez-Máximo JD, et al. Dimensions of community assets for health. A systematised review and meta-synthesis. Int J Environ Res Public Health. 2021;18:18.

Sanders Thompson VL, Ackermann N, Bauer KL, Bowen DJ, Goodman MS. Strategies of community engagement in research: definitions and classifications. Transl Behav Med. 2021;11(2):441–51. https://doi.org/10.1093/tbm/ibaa042

Sandmann LR, Watkins KE. Action technologies: contemporary community-engaged action research. In: Knox AB, Conceição SCO, Martin LG, Glowacki-Dudka M, Mott VW, Tennant M, et al., editors. Mapping the field of adult and continuing education. 1st ed. Routledge; 2017. p. 629–35.

Santos BS. The end of the cognitive empire: the coming of age of epistemologies of the south. 1st ed. Durham: Duke University Press; 2018.

Senge PM. The fifth discipline: the art and practice of the learning organization. Rev and updated. London: Random House Business; 2006.

Smith LT. Decolonizing methodologies: research and indigenous peoples. Third; 1;3;Third. London: Zed; 2021.

Sofolahan-Oladeinde Y, Mullins CD, Baquet CR. Using community-based participatory research in patient-centered outcomes research to address health disparities in under-represented communities. J Comp Eff Res. 2015;4(5):515–23.

Stein A, Dainels J, Fields CD, Palmer N, editors. Going public: a guide for social scientists 2017.

Stilgoe J, Lock SJ, Wilsdon J. Why should we promote public engagement with science? Public Underst Sci. 2014;23(1):4–15.

Trencher GP, Bai X, Evans J, McCormick K, Yarime M. University partnerships for co-designing and co-producing urban sustainability. Global Environ Change Human Policy Dimensions. 2014a;28:153–65.

Trencher GP, Yarime M, McCormick K, Doll C, Kraines SB. Beyond the third mission: exploring the emerging university function of co-creation for sustainability. Sci Public Policy. 2014b;41:151–79.

Van De Ven AH, Johnson PE. Knowledge for theory and practice. Acad Manag Rev. 2006;31(4):802–21.

Vicente-Saez R, Martínez-Fuentes C. Open Science now: a systematic literature review for an integrated definition. J Bus Res. 2018;88:428.

Wallerstein N, Duran B. Community-based participatory research contributions to intervention research: the intersection of science and practice to improve health equity. Am J Public Health. 2010;100(Suppl 1):S40–6.

Wallerstein N, Wallerstein N, Giatti LL, Giatti LL, Bógus CM, Bógus CM, et al. Shared participatory research principles and methodologies: perspectives from the USA and Brazil—45 years after Paulo Freire's "pedagogy of the oppressed". Societies. 2017;7(2):6.

Watermeyer R. Issues in the articulation of 'impact': the responses of UK academics to 'impact' as a new measure of research assessment. Stud High Educ (Dorchester-on-Thames). 2014;39(2):359–77.

Watermeyer R, Chubb J. Evaluating 'impact' in the UK's research excellence framework (REF): liminality, looseness and new modalities of scholarly distinction. Stud High Educ. 2019;44:1554–66.

Watson D, Hollister R, Stroud SE, Babcock E. The engaged university: international perspectives on civic engagement. In: International studies in higher education. Routledge, Taylor & Francis Group; 2011.

Chapter 2
Building the Engaged Research Ecosystem

2.1 Introduction

Engaged research, characterised by active collaboration between researchers and community stakeholders, is paramount for research performing organisations (RPOs) aiming to generate impactful and socially relevant knowledge (Bednarek and Tseng 2022). This approach not only enhances the quality and applicability of research outcomes by integrating diverse perspectives and expertise but also fosters trust and mutual respect between academia and the public. Engaged research facilitates the co-creation of solutions to complex societal challenges, ensuring that research agendas align with community needs and priorities. Moreover, it enhances the dissemination and implementation of research findings, thereby maximising their societal impact and contributing to the overall mission of RPOs to advance knowledge and foster innovation for the public good.

Traditional approaches to research, often characterised by a top-down methodology and a primary focus on academic outputs, have inadvertently resulted in legacy and capacity issues for engaged research (Burgwal and van de Burgwal 2018). These conventional methods frequently prioritise the advancement of theoretical knowledge over practical applications, leading to a disconnect between researchers and the communities they study. Consequently, research agendas and outcomes may lack relevance to real-world problems, diminishing the potential for meaningful community impact. Additionally, the absence of collaborative frameworks and stakeholder involvement in traditional research practices has limited the development of skills and capacities necessary for effective engagement. This has perpetuated a cycle where both researchers and communities are ill-prepared for genuine co-creation processes, further entrenching the divide between academic research and societal needs (Mallonee et al. 2006; Polk 2014). Addressing these legacy issues requires a paradigm shift towards inclusive and participatory research models that prioritise capacity building and foster enduring partnerships.

E. R. Dorris et al., *Building the Ecosystem for Engaged Research*,
SpringerBriefs in Public Health, https://doi.org/10.1007/978-3-031-82080-9_2

Reactive and proactive approaches to engaged research represent two distinct strategies for integrating community involvement in the research process. Reactive approaches typically respond to immediate issues or crises, involving stakeholders and communities after problems have emerged (Heiner et al. 2019). This method, while beneficial in addressing urgent needs, often results in short-term solutions and limited long-term impact. Reactive engagement can sometimes reinforce power imbalances, as communities may feel their input is sought only during times of crisis rather than as part of a continuous dialogue.

In contrast, proactive approaches emphasise ongoing, forward-thinking collaboration between researchers and stakeholders. This strategy involves building long-term relationships, identifying potential issues before they arise, and co-developing research agendas that reflect community priorities from the outset. Proactive engagement fosters trust, mutual respect, and shared ownership of research processes and outcomes. It enhances the capacity of both researchers and communities to address complex, evolving challenges and ensures that research efforts are relevant, sustainable, and impactful. By adopting a proactive approach, research performing organizations can create more resilient and adaptive research ecosystems, ultimately leading to more effective and inclusive solutions to societal problems.

Investing in proactive approaches to engaged research is crucial for RPOs to remain relevant and effective in addressing contemporary societal challenges. By fostering continuous, forward-looking collaboration with communities, RPOs can anticipate and mitigate emerging issues, rather than merely reacting to them. This investment not only enhances the societal relevance and impact of research but also builds stronger, more resilient partnerships with stakeholders (Saunders 2022). Furthermore, proactive engagement promotes inclusivity and equity in the research process, ensuring diverse voices are heard and integrated into the development of solutions (Goulden and Morrison 2022). Such an approach strengthens the credibility and trustworthiness of RPOs, positioning them as leaders in producing research that truly serves the public good.

This chapter will focus on how RPOs can adapt, foster, and support a proactive approach to engaged research. It will focus on the institutional ecosystem, rather than individual or project level approaches.

2.2 Reforms to Research Funding

Traditional research funding models, which often prioritise outputs such as publications, patents, and high-impact discoveries, can be misaligned with the principles and practices of engaged research. These conventional funding frameworks typically emphasise short-term project cycles, measurable deliverables, and competitive grant mechanisms, which may not provide the necessary flexibility and timeframes required for meaningful community collaboration and long-term engagement.

Engaged research, by its nature, involves iterative processes, relationship building, and the co-creation of knowledge, all of which require sustained investment and support beyond typical funding cycles (Edwards and Edwards 2017). Furthermore, traditional funding models often lack mechanisms to adequately value and support the participatory elements of engaged research, such as community consultation, capacity building, and dissemination of findings in accessible formats.

As a result, researchers committed to engaged practices may struggle to secure funding, limiting their ability to pursue collaborative projects that address community needs. To be effective, funding models must evolve to recognise and support the unique demands of engaged research. This includes providing longer-term grants, encouraging interdisciplinary collaboration, and valuing diverse types of outputs and impacts that extend beyond traditional academic metrics. Adapting funding mechanisms in this way is essential to foster a research environment where engaged practices can thrive and deliver significant societal benefits.

To support engaged research effectively, research funders can implement several key improvements that align funding mechanisms with the unique demands and benefits of this collaborative approach. First, extending the duration of grants can provide the necessary time for building and maintaining meaningful relationships with community stakeholders. Long-term funding commitments allow for iterative cycles of feedback, adaptation, and co-creation, essential for addressing complex societal issues.

Example: The Wellcome Trust Model
In 2010 the Wellcome Trust, an independent charitable foundation that funds health research, changed their funding model to fund people rather than projects. This change came with a longer funding period (average of 7 years) and greater freedom and flexibility to pursue their research vision rather than solely pursuing project deliverables. In their 2021 strategy, although they made many changes, they maintained the flexibility and longer duration of funding (between 5 and 8 years, with an option for longer for those working part-time). This longer duration is to allow researchers to focus on innovative and impactful research rather than constantly having to apply for grants. The Wellcome Trust also actively encourages an engaged research approach as they "believe using an engaged research approach improves research and makes it more impactful". (Wellcome Trust 2024)

Funders can introduce flexible funding models that accommodate the diverse activities involved in engaged research. This includes allocating resources for community consultation, capacity building, and the dissemination of findings in formats accessible to non-academic audiences. Recognising and valuing these activities in funding criteria will encourage researchers to prioritise genuine engagement.

Example: SFI and Irish Aid SDG Challenge
Science Foundation Ireland (SFI, a public agency responsible for funding oriented basic and applied research) and Irish Aid (the Government of Ireland's international development aid programme) have solution-orientated SDG challenge funding. Each project team must have a societal impact champion "to provide non-technical leadership and support to identify and validate challenges, in addition to advising on solution development". The funding is provided in phases. The concept phase is funded for 6 months to form and establish a societally impactful research team. There is a dedicated budget which will allow relevant consultations and engagement to understand the local context and feasibility of proposed solution-oriented research. Building in this phase provides the funding and resources necessary to engage with the necessary stakeholders and societal actors relevant to the downstream phases of the research. (SFI 2024)

Interdisciplinary and cross-sector collaboration should be incentivised, as engaged research often requires integrating knowledge and expertise from various fields. Funders can establish special grants or collaborative platforms that bring together academic researchers, community organisations, and industry partners to address shared challenges.

Example: The European Citizen Science Platform
The European citizen science platform is an EU-funded action to build capacity for citizen science and promote societal change in Europe. This acts as a knowledge hub for people, projects, education, and resources related to citizen science to be found and shared. This is an investment that is being built upon in iterative projects such as the EU-funded European Citizen Science project which is expanding the platform to a global reach (EU Citizen Science 2024).

Additionally, funders can incorporate criteria that assess the societal impact and relevance of research proposals, alongside traditional academic metrics. This shift in evaluation can highlight the importance of community engagement and the co-production of knowledge, rewarding projects that demonstrate clear benefits to society.

> **Example: Health Research Board Public Reviewers**
> The Health Research Board (HRB) is a government agency responsible for funding health research in Ireland. Public and patient involvement (PPI) in research has been part of its research strategy since 2016. In 2017 it sought interest from members of the public to review specific aspects of research proposals submitted to the HRB. Initially, the public reviews were used solely to provide direct feedback to applicant teams so teams could integrate that feedback thereby gaining experience of incorporating public and patient involvement (PPI) into their research proposals. In 2020, they integrated the public reviews into the HRB funding decisions. The HRB is continuing to iteratively progress both how they support PPI in their processes and how they encourage researchers they fund to do the same. (HRB n.d., 2021)

By implementing these improvements, research funders can create an environment that supports and values engaged research, ultimately leading to more impactful and socially relevant outcomes. However, the onus is not solely on research funders to improve the ecosystem for engaged research. RPOs also need to adapt to the evolving landscape and actively make improvements to support the environment required for sustainable engaged research.

2.3   Evolving Research Supports

Traditional research support services are not designed with engaged research approaches in mind. Embracing engaged research requires each of the supporting research units of an RPO to be aware of the different needs, and indeed goals, of engaged research. Without a joined up and embedded approach, the procedures and systems of an RPO can cause frustration that hinders progress (Maccarthy et al. 2019). The addition of engaged research personnel can only progress the ecosystem so much, without reforms across the supporting structure.

Pre-award services, defined as the support unit(s) responsible for identifying and disseminating funding opportunities, submitting applications, and reviewing applications, will need to be made aware of the changing landscape. There can be aspects of engaged research funding proposals that differ from traditional proposal. For example, a need to front load grant budgets for relationship and collaboration building and designing digital or analogue tools supportive of such. Some of the external co-applicants may not have access to the typical training and writing supports of traditional co-applicants. Pre-award units will need to decide if and when these external societal partners will receive support in the preparation of their parts of a grant proposal, and if so, how that additional labour will be resourced. If they are to be able to assist with proposals, pre-award staff should be supported by access to experienced engaged research personnel or resources that highlight good practices for engaged research. This can include identifying what an enabling budget and budget justification looks like, identifying elements of engaged research throughout the entire project and project management plan, and being able to identify the added value of collaboration within engaged research funding proposals.

Grant registration and contract support units can benefit from understanding the issues and creating potential solutions for societal organisations with limited capacity. External partners funded through a grant award are typically set up as subcontractors. Ensuring that information like this is communicated at proposal preparation can help to ensure that societal partners who are listed as funded investigators have the capacity to legally undertake the subcontract. This can prevent downstream delays in the execution of contracts for the funding award. This unit(s) can also produce standard templates with the legal clauses explained in order to assist societal partners with limited capacity or access to legal expertise. However, these RPO units are also limited in the support they can provide to external partners because independent legal advice is part of best practice under contract law (MacMillan 2022). The RPO cannot be perceived to have circumvented the external partner seeking, or their perceived opportunity to seek, independent legal advice prior to executing the contract.

Finance and human resources are both important units to support sustainable engaged research. These units are typically responsible for policy and procedures related to remittance and payment of engaged research contributors. Safety and insurance units may also need to be involved in ensuring appropriate insurance or indemnification of those involved in engaged research. If a research collaboration is being undertaken, it is generally considered that it is morally wrong to have the societal partner as the only unpaid member(s) of a consortium. However, there is often a lack of a process or policy on how to remunerate people in a standardised and fiscally compliant manner (Richards et al. 2022). For sustainable practice of engaged research this is one of the most important hurdles to overcome. Both HR and finance need to be informed of the scope and scale of engaged research practices happening at an RPO. This can help them to understand the regulatory and potential fiscal and tax compliance needs for the development of a sustainable remittance policy for engaged research contributors.

Engaged research often has a focus on co-creation of knowledge and products. This has led to the need for consideration of non-traditional intellectual property (IP) and licensing pathways (Tekic and Willoughby 2020). Co-creation can blur the boundaries of IP ownership (Tekic et al. 2023). The creation of the IP must be documented meticulously, including detailed records of development, dates, and contributions. Clear agreements and contracts are typically necessary, especially in collaborative environments, to delineate ownership rights and ensure that all contributors' roles are legally acknowledged. However, in a setting where the partners may not have the legal knowledge or support to understand their potential ownership rights, how can these issues be fairly and equitably addressed? To uphold ownership and value, the IP must be maintained and defended through regular renewals, monitoring for infringements, and enforcing rights through litigation if necessary. These are essential ongoing processes. When the funding for the project has lapsed, RPOs may carry out these ongoing processes on behalf of their researchers (RPOs often at least co-own the assets). But how can less formal societal partners access the funding and expertise required for these ongoing processes beyond the funding lifecycle? While it is not a direct responsibility of the RPO to solve this, it certainly would stand to their benefit to contribute to finding solutions if they are seeking ongoing engagement with diverse societal partners. Having plain English guidance and templates where collaborations can outline each partner's expected creation, contribution, and any pre-existing legal registrations in advance of working together may help downstream to define who holds the rights to use, sell, or license the intellectual property.

> **Example: The New Toolbox for Sustainable IP Licensing**
> IMPAC3T-IP is an EU-funded action that is addressing scenario-based licensing for stakeholders in the IP value chain. The project is developing a toolbox and an associated training programme to support licensing in non-traditional scenarios, including co-creation. This programme addresses critical challenges highlighted by the European Commission's Action Plan on Intellectual Property. Its aim is to accelerate socially responsible IP management processes in diverse scenarios, including when IP is created by complex partnerships with multiple owners and diverse licensing objectives. RPOs should follow the output of this action for emerging processes and guidance on managing IP in these more complex scenarios. (IMPAC3T-IP 2024)

2.4 Infrastructure to Sustain Engaged Research

2.4.1 Training

To support engaged research effectively, RPOs can establish a comprehensive training infrastructure that equips researchers and engaged research partners with the necessary skills and knowledge. This infrastructure should include various components designed to foster engagement, collaboration, and capacity building. Engaged research is based on the concept of multi-stakeholder collaboration (Holliman 2017). Many of the necessary core concepts may already exist within the RPO's research and innovation training catalogue but need to be adapted for an engaged research lens. For example, communication skills, including effective communication strategies and public speaking, may already exist. Similarly, conflict resolution and negotiation for productive and respectful collaborations may already be within an RPOs innovation arm. Co-production with engaged research partners to adapt these trainings and resources can make repurposing these trainings cost-effective and time-saving for RPOs.

RPOs can offer or financially support workshops, mentorship programmes, and resources to help researchers navigate the complexities of collaborative work with external stakeholders (Guerrini et al. 2018). There is an argument that RPOs should also be at least partially responsible for providing learning and upskilling for engaged research partners in addition to RPO staff (Holliman and Warren 2017). RPOs have expertise that can be used for capacity building for engaged research partners. This may include offering training to engaged research partners that helps them better understand research processes, research skills that may be applicable to them, and effective collaboration techniques.

E-learning platforms with online courses and tutorials on engaged research can be particularly useful as engaged research partners can be diverse in their availability.

RPOs should support mutual learning approaches, where RPO staff, researchers, and community partners learn from each other's perspectives and expertise. RPOs can support this through supportive funding and use of RPO meeting spaces.

Establishing recognition processes for engaged research training programmes, such as digital badges, credits (for postgraduate students or continuous professional development), or certification programmes, can formally recognise and validate the skills and knowledge of researchers. This can make training a more attractive offering to target learners (Kafaji 2020). Training for engaged research is often co-delivered by experienced engaged research partner. RPOs should have processes in place for payment of the partner, be that via occasional guest lecturer or adjunct lecturer. The criteria for expertise required for these roles should be adapted to include lived experience in this context.

2.4.2   Centralised Resources

In many research disciplines, engaged research and engaged research practices are not new. The terminology popular in current parlance may be different, but the underlying concepts of stakeholder and community engagement, involvement, and participation have long been central to certain research disciplines (see Chap. 1). From an RPO perspective, one of the issues is research knowledge being held in silos, but this is also one of the biggest opportunities. Investing in centralising and developing centralised resources for engaged research can help to capture and share the existing knowledge within the RPO's community. Centralised resources often result in improved communication and coordination because the central point acts as a hub for information flow (Andrews et al. 2017). Centralisation supports more equitable access and allows the whole community to leverage collective knowledge and best practices. This can spur innovation and continuous improvement across an RPO.

Centralising engaged research resources can foster an environment where knowledge sharing is encouraged. It also provides a space to increase visibility of those using engaged research approaches. An often stated perception amongst researchers is that traditional RPO systems do not champion those who take time to foster relationships and collaboration for societal benefit. Having an RPO-level dedicated centralised space reinforces the institutional commitment to engaged research and is an outward demonstration of the underpinning infrastructure supportive of engaged research.

From an RPO's perspective, centralisation enables better monitoring and management of engaged research needs (Ryttberg and Geschwind 2021). Using analytics to identify which resources are accessed most frequently and which are the most frequently asked questions enables more strategic and effective development and deployment of engaged research supports and helps with sustainability planning. This can ensure that resources are used optimally and aligned with the RPO's overarching goals.

2.4.3   Digital Infrastructure

Supporting engaged research requires robust digital infrastructure that facilitates communication, collaboration, data management, and dissemination among researchers, community stakeholders, and other partners. Key components of this infrastructure are discussed below.

2.4.3.1   Collaboration Platforms

There are many existing collaboration platforms available. However, issues can arise around the openness of those platforms. Engaged research is collaborative by nature and therefore internal or staff options are not viable. Consideration needs to be given to who has access to online collaboration tools and virtual meeting software to facilitate real-time communication and project management. There is a financial impact for access, training, and maintenance of these systems for external partners. When external partners are charitable and community organisations, or members of the public contributing to research and development, the expectation is that RPOs will be responsible for those costs. This needs to be considered when RPOs are budgeting for these systems.

2.4.3.2   Community Engagement Portals

Researchers and engaged research partners require mechanisms to identify each other and interact. Digital mechanisms to facilitate this are growing. These can range from social media integration which leverages social media platforms to disseminate information, gather feedback, and engage with broader audiences in a more informal setting. These can be easier to implement, especially when RPOs have clear social media guidelines.

These are also interactive websites with features, such as forums, individual or group profiles, networking options, and feedback mechanisms. These can be particularly useful for research with a larger network of engaged research partners (Leipämaa-Leskinen et al. 2022). However, these are often on a project-specific basis which is not sustainable as they depend on the availability of project funding and can become defunct post-project lifecycle when funding runs out. This represents research waste and can also lead to frustration in the engaged research partners who may need to learn different systems for different projects. There is scope for RPO or governmental level maintenance of community engagement portals.

> **Example: Flemish Knowledge Centre for Citizen Science**
> Scivil is the Flemish knowledge Centre for citizen science of the Flanders region of Belgium. Scivil operates as a public initiative, working in collaboration with various stakeholders including universities, research institutions, governmental bodies, and civil society organisations. The aim is to foster and support citizen science across the region rather than to generate profit or serve the interests of private owners. It bridges the gap between professional researchers and the general public through providing resources, training, and networking opportunities. Scivil enables engagement and collaboration among different stakeholders, including academic institutions, government agencies, non-profit organisations, and the public. It is generally acknowledged that Scivil has helped build a stronger, more cohesive citizen science community in Flanders. (Scivil n.d.)

2.4.3.3 Data Management Systems

All research requires secure data repositories and engaged research is no different. Cloud-based storage solutions like institutional repositories provide secure and data storage accessible to RPO members. However, can these repositories be accessed by engaged research partners in a manner that ensures that research data can be shared and managed collaboratively? Processes need to be put in place to ensure access while maintaining security.

There are existing tools that facilitate the sharing of research data with engaged research partners while maintaining privacy and security standards. Data sharing platforms such as Figshare (https://figshare.com/), Zenodo (https://zenodo.org/), and Open Science Framework (OSF) (https://osf.io/) may be viable existing options for engaged research at RPOs. RPOs can implement institutional level guidelines or policies for the permissible use of such external platforms.

2.4.3.4 Security and Privacy Infrastructure

Attention needs to be given to ensuring engaged research partners have the digital capacity required for encryption technologies and robust access control mechanisms. It cannot be assumed that engaged research partners, which may include individuals in their personal capacity, have encryption and access control compliance management tools (Barony Sanchez et al. 2022). Therefore, there must be active steps taken to ensure all partners have the digital hardware and software necessary for research integrity and data protection regulations.

2.4.4 Personnel

To effectively support engaged research at RPOs, dedicated personnel with specific roles and responsibilities are an important investment. At project level, engaged research personnel bridge the gap between academic research and community needs, ensuring that collaborative projects are both impactful and sustainable. As outlined in Fig. 2.1, embedding engaged research needs to happen across systems at institutional level. Managing the implementation of this requires specific skill sets, which can be different from that of project staff managing community-researcher interactions.

Engaged research staff working to embed institutional change and supports need to understand change management, multi-stakeholder management, and have an ability to understand, influence, and implement engaged research policy. They are "knowledge managers and brokers" among internal and external stakeholders. Their work requires a particular understanding and skill sets, characterised by openness, empathy, trust building, creativity, and management expertise.

2.5 Monitoring and Evaluation

Engaged research can bring many benefits but does require investment from RPOs. As per any investment, there should be infrastructure put in place to allow the monitoring and evaluation of engaged research. However, standardised metrics that can be implemented at an institutional level are difficult to identify and define given the nature and intent of engaged research. There is a general consensus that engaged research should be evaluated (Table 2.1); however, the identification of metrics to do so in a meaningful way is less clear. In order for RPOs to develop useful comprehensive evaluation frameworks, these frameworks need clear criteria and metrics that capture the complexity of engagement outcomes and impact.

At project level, there is more scope for the use of comprehensive evaluation frameworks tailored to the specific goals and context of engaged research. Recent publications, such as the independent report from the European Commission, discuss in depth measuring the value of engaged research based on an analysis of 60 research projects (European Commission et al. 2024). It recommends 12 potential key performance indicators across the dimensions of outreach, participatory activities, and value creation. However, while very welcome for the research community, there is still a gap in knowledge as to how to best evaluate engaged research institutionally. A harmonised approach to monitoring and evaluation of engaged research has yet to be defined. However, in Table 2.1 and the discussion below, we highlight potential processes and indicators that could be included as part of an RPO's engaged research evaluation framework.

United Kingdom Research and Innovation (UKRI) is a non-departmental public body of the UK Government. They developed robust and iterative frameworks for evaluation excellence of both research and knowledge exchange across higher

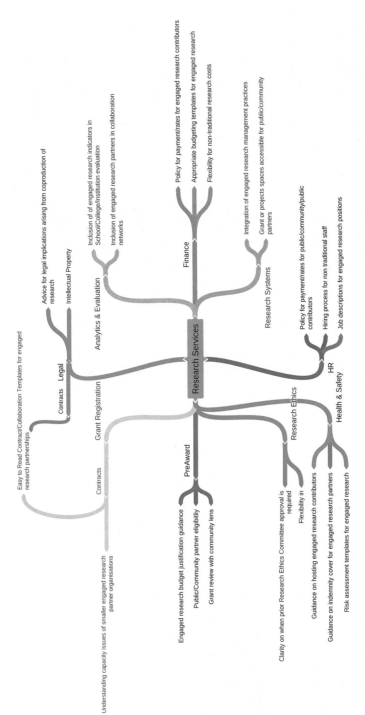

Fig. 2.1 Integration of engaged research requires a systems approach. Branches represent research support units. Examples of how they are important for embedding engaged research are listed at the end of each branch

Table 2.1 Engaged research metrics and indicators from key national and international frameworks. Y=Yes; N=No; R=Recommended; P=Project level

Name	Affiliation	Publisher (Country)	R&D	Project level	Institutional level	Metrics or indicators	Notes	Discipline specific	Reference
CIHR'S citizen engagement handbook	Canadian Institutes of Health Research (CIHR)	Canada	Y	Y	N	Y	Process evaluation and outcome indicators	Y	CIHR (2012)
Community engagement framework for quality, people-centred, and resilient health services	World Health Organization (WHO)	Switzerland	N	N	Y	R	"It is important to establish platforms for the monitoring and reporting of activities and indicators of success; to engage community members in monitoring and reporting activities and in systematically reflecting on the data and what it means; to develop feedback mechanisms that use qualitative andquantitative data to help key stakeholders effectively engage with each other and contribute to a coherent and informed response; and to ensure transparency and available, timely data on progress and impact, that is tailored to multiple stakeholders" pg. 24	Y	WHO (2017)
Engaged research framework	Irish universities association	Ireland	Y	Y	N	P	Provides categories and reflective questions to consider for impact assessment (p9)	N	Bowman et al. (2022)

(continued)

Table 2.1 (continued)

Name	Affiliation	Publisher (Country)	R&D	Project level	Institutional level	Metrics or indicators	Notes	Discipline specific	Reference
Fostering knowledge valorisation through citizen engagement	EU Commission	Belgium	Y	Y	N	Y	Annex 3: list of proposed indicators	N	European Commission (2024)
Minimum quality standards and indicators for community engagement	UNICEF	USA	Partial	N	Y	Y	p. 36 these indicators are not designed for universal adoption, and there are no current expectations for mandatory reporting. Institutions have their own needs and requirements and can use these indicators as a starting point for launching organisation-specific initiatives to design monitoring and evaluation processes, measurement approaches, and methodologies that are fit for purpose and context specific.	N	UNICEF (2020)

Title	Organisation	Country					Description		Reference
Strategic framework for mainstreaming citizen engagement in World Bank Group operations: Engaging with citizens for improved results	World Bank	USA	N	*	*	P	Not research indicators. p.114 propose to creation of a list of sector agnostic CE indicators	Y	Hamad et al. (2014)
The code of practice on citizen engagement for knowledge valorisation	EU Commission	Belgium	Y	Y	Y	R	2.8. It is recommended to adopt at organisational level a clearly defined evaluation framework to assess the efficacy of citizen engagement and participatory processes that lead to knowledge valorisation	N	European Commission (2024)
UK standards for public involvement	NIHR, CSO (Scotland), health and care research Wales and the PHA (northern Ireland)	UK	Y	Y	Y	Partial	Each standard has a "meeting the standard" guidance	Y	NIHR et al. (2018)

education institutions (HEIs) in the United Kingdom (UKRI 2024a). Public and community engagement and research partnerships are included in the Knowledge Exchange Framework (KEF, UKRI 2024b). Research partnership has two metrics. The first is the financial contribution to collaborative research as a proportion of public funding. The data for this research is collected as part of the UK Higher Education Business and Community Interaction (HE-BCI) survey, which collects financial and output data related to knowledge exchange in the United Kingdom each academic year (see Chap. 4). Modelling this metric in other regions would require similar government level investment to collect the relevant data in a standardised process across research active HEIs.

The second research partnership metric used in the KEF is co-authorship with non-academic partners as a proportion of total outputs. The data for this metric at UKRI is provided by the research analytics and data service provider Elsevier. Many RPOs already have infrastructure in place to implement this metric, such as a subscription to research analytic service providers and in-house output analytic skills. Thus, in well-funded RPOs such as western HEIs, this may be a usable metric to model. This metric would not be sufficient in and of itself to measure engaged research but could act as a supportive metric to benchmark outputs with non-academic authors against similar institutions.

Public and community engagement evaluation is optional for inclusion in the KEF. This section is not limited to research, but more broadly focused on how HEIs interact with the community in a mutually beneficial way. The KEF uses a narrative statement approach, with each institution self-assessing how well they believe they are doing against defined scoring criteria (UKRI 2024b). It is not externally scored. It has five aspects that cover public and community engagement in HEI strategy through delivery of strategy goals and monitoring and evaluation of such. This reinforces the need to consider whole-system support for public and community engagement. This format gives flexibility to HEIs in their approach to community and public engagement. It is more labour intensive and relies on infrastructure that can collect qualitative narratives underpinned by supportive evidence. If RPOs have sufficient personnel, skills, and processes to capture this evidence, the structure may be a useful model. However, unless it is being used internally only or as one part of larger evaluation based on scoring (as per the KEF), it is questionable how much benefit the subjective self-assessment scores provide. It is well known that self-assessment scores demonstrate relatively low reliability. If the goal of the narrative statement is reflective practice for quality improvement, the use of arbitrary "scoring" could detract from achieving this goal.

UNICEF developed minimum standards and indicators for community engagement (UNICEF 2020). They are not research specific, but rather provide guidance for community engagement in high-, middle-, and low-income countries across all sectors. There are 16 standards across 4 categories (core standards, implementation, coordination and integration, and resource mobilisation) and suggested indicators for each standard. Core standards and implementation are largely project focused, whereas coordination and integration are predominantly government focused. From an RPO perspective, the resource mobilisation category is the most relevant, as it refers to the management and administrative functions that support community engagement activities and systems. There are a variety of indicators suggested as potential ways to assess if the minimum standards are being achieved. The standards in the resource mobilisation category are: human resources and organisational structure (standard 14), data management (standard 15), and resource mobilisation and budgeting (standard 16). The recommended indicators have an associated Likert scale to measure progress towards an enabling environment. Like the KEF self-narrative assessment, the intention is to measure progress in embedding of an environment supportive of community engagement, rather as a comparative measure against other institutions. The range of indicators is provided so institutions can select those most appropriate to their individual context. Whereas the indicators as listed in the UNICEF publication may not be directly transferable into the research context, minor adaptations can make them useful for monitoring progress in RPOs. These indicators tend to be less labour intense to collect comparatively to the public and community engagement narrative.

2.6   Complexity and Tensions of Implementing Engaged Research

This chapter has discussed the reform and change required in RPOs to facilitate a culture of engaged research. Institutional strategies, however, are not always aligned with the underlying value proposition of engaged research. Engaged research often focuses on the democratisation of the research process and co-ownership of solutions with communities. In RPOs where rankings, metrics, and indicators include the number of RPO-led patents, spin-out companies, and investment in RPO-led projects, there is an inherent tension. The RPO must demonstrate innovation and excellence by leading impactful projects, yet engaged research often advocates for the co-creation of research and shared ownership of intellectual property (Szluka et al. 2023). This can dilute the current metrics used by RPOs to demonstrate innovation and research excellence. A wider sea change in the culture of how we value and measure research excellence always needs to be part of the conversation when discussing engaged research (Gerke et al. 2023). Measuring societal impact of social innovations is much trickier and labour intensive than measuring in patent or investment numbers (Reed 2016). Until this issue of assessment and measurement is solved, a tension will remain within RPOs.

An RPO's legacy may also hinder engaged research. Some RPOs, especially older universities or research institutes based on historical endowments, have a legacy of colonialism, imperialism, and religious affiliation embedded within their history that can significantly hinder their efforts toward meaningful community engagement (Yep and Mitchell 2017). Such a legacy often perpetuates structures of privilege and exclusion that align the institution with past injustices, rendering it difficult for some communities to view the RPO as a genuine partner in addressing contemporary social issues. Historical affiliations may lead to mistrust, scepticism, and resistance from communities who feel that their identities, experiences, and needs are not adequately represented or respected, thereby obstructing the development of equitable and collaborative partnerships essential for effective community engagement. Addressing historical wrongs involves navigating complex challenges and divergent expectations that can be uncomfortable for institutions accustomed to projecting an image of authority and moral leadership (Merchant et al. 2014). However, there has been an increase in institutions undergoing critical re-evaluation of their history, acknowledging and confronting past injustices and their ongoing impacts on certain communities (Shahid and McGee 2021). Through examining and reforming governance structures and policies to ensure they are inclusive and representative of the broader community and committing to transparency, accountability, and sustained efforts to redress historical wrongs, institutions can begin to rebuild trust and foster more authentic, equitable relationships with the communities they serve. Any type of legacy issue requires time and effort to rebuild trust with a community.

This book focuses on RPOs, particularly research performing higher education institutions. However, RPOs are only one member of an engaged research partnership. Much of this chapter has assumed that RPOs will be the leading institution in a research project. This is an example of the implicit assumptions of power that is common in research. Power and perceived power arise from who has the formal authority to make decisions and who controls resources (Dorris 2024). In addition, there are fewer tangible aspects to power such as the ability to control ideas and meaning. RPO-led research is still the norm; user-led research is gaining traction. There are multiple ways in which user-led research is being implemented. Research charities are hiring researchers to carry out research directly, research prioritisation within communities is being used as the criteria for funding calls, and end users are being included in peer review of funding applications. However, user-led research also needs to be supported. Lack of capacity in the community sector is frequently identified as a barrier to greater involvement in research. Who is responsible for providing that support, for upskilling and acquiring the foundational knowledge of good research practice?

2.7   Summary and Key Messages

Engaging the public in research can provide a number of benefits to research, researchers, and research organisations in addition to societal benefits. However, an integrated approach needs to be developed in order to institutionally embed engaged research practices in a sustainable manner. Engaged research is a change in approach to research, and therefore requires change across the entire research ecosystem. Embedding this approach in RPOs requires change across research support units and buy-in from the highest levels of management downwards. There needs to be institutional acknowledgement that engaged research is not just a "nice thing to do" but a fundamental need to maximising the potential societal impact of research.

Key Messages
1. The responsibility for creating a sustainable ecosystem of engaged research lies with multiple research stakeholders including RPOs, policymakers, public authorities, and civil society.
2. Research funders can learn from each other in how to innovate funding mechanisms to be more supportive of engaged research.
3. RPOs need to take a system-wide approach to supporting engaged research to ensure sustainability.
4. Monitoring and evaluation of engaged research is important to build up the evidence base for these approaches. While many frameworks recommend institutional-level evaluation, most of the existing indicators are project level and unsuitable for use institutionally.

References

Andrews R, Boyne G, Mostafa AMS. When bureaucracy matters for organizational performance: exploring the benefits of administrative intensity in big and complex organizations. Public Adm. 2017;95(1):115–39.

Barony Sanchez RH, Bergeron-Drolet LA, Sasseville M, Gagnon MP. Engaging patients and citizens in digital health technology development through the virtual space. Front Med Technol. 2022;4:958571.

Bednarek A, Tseng V. A global movement for engaged research. Issues Sci Technol. 2022;38(3):53–6.

Bowman S, Morris K, O'Neill D, Foley C, Cody A, Bates C, et al. A framework for engaged research 2022.. 2024. Available from: https://www.iua.ie/wp-content/uploads/2023/12/Guide-IUA-Engaged-Research-Framework-2022_V7-11.pdf

Burgwal LVD, van de Burgwal LHM. On the societal impact of knowledge: understanding knowledge valorisation in the life sciences. 2018.

CIHR. CIHR's citizen engagement handbook 2012. 2024. Available from: https://cihr-irsc.gc.ca/e/42196.html

Dorris E. Improving impact: public involvement in glycobiology research. In: Kilcoyne M, Joshi L, editors. Translational Glycobiology in human health and disease. Academic Press; 2024. p. 399–419.

Edwards K, Edwards KE. Engaged research and practice: higher education and the pursuit of the public good. Partnerships J Serv Learn Civic Engag. 2017;8(1):47–9.

European Citizen Science. European citizen science platform 2024.. Available from: https://eu-citizen.science/

European Commission: Directorate-General for R, Innovation. Valorisation policies—code of practice on citizen engagement—commission recommendation: Publications Office of the European Union; 2024.

European Commission: Directorate-General for R, Innovation, Pottaki I, Monaco F, Articolo R, Martinez E, et al. Fostering knowledge valorisation through citizen engagement. Publications Office of the European Union; 2024.

Gerke D-M, Uude K, Kliewe T. Co-creation and societal impact: toward a generic framework for research impact assessment. Evaluation. 2023;29:489–508.

Goulden H, Morrison E. An equitable future for research and innovation. The Young Foundation; 2022.

Guerrini CJ, Majumder MA, Lewellyn MJ, McGuire AL. Citizen science, public policy. Science. 2018;361(6398):134.

Hamad QHU, Zenaida; Mahmood, Syed A.; Manroth, Astrid; Masud, Harika; Peixoto, Tiago Carneiro; Rebolledo Dellepiane, Miguel Angel; Seyedian, Aaron; Zakhour, Jad Karim. Strategic framework for mainstreaming citizen engagement in World Bank Group operations: engaging with citizens for improved results (English). 2014.. Available from: http://documents.worldbank.org/curated/en/266371468124780089/Strategic-framework-for-mainstreaming-citizen-engagement-in-World-Bank-Group-operations-engaging-with-citizens-for-improved-results

Heiner M, Hinchley D, Fitzsimons J, Weisenberger F, Bergmann W, McMahon T, et al. Moving from reactive to proactive development planning to conserve indigenous community and biodiversity values. Environ Impact Assess Rev. 2019;74:1–13.

Holliman R. Supporting excellence in engaged research. J Sci Commun. 2017;16(5):1–10.

Holliman R, Warren CJ, editors. Supporting future scholars of engaged research. Res ALL. 2017;1(1):168–84.

HRB. HRB strategy 2021–2025: health research - making an impact. Dublin: Health Research Board; 2021.

HRB. How we assess applications Dublin: Health Research Board.. Available from: https://www.hrb.ie/funding/funding-opportunities/how-we-assess-applications/. n.d.

IMPAC3T-IP. The new toolbox for sustainable IP licensing 2024. Available from: https://www.impac3tip.eu/

Kafaji M. The perceived benefits of accreditation on students' performance: the case of private business schools. Ind High Educ. 2020;34(6):421–8.

Leipämaa-Leskinen H, Närvänen E, Makkonen H. The rise of collaborative engagement platforms. Eur J Mark. 2022;56(13):26–49.

Maccarthy J, Guerin S, Wilson AG, Dorris ER. Facilitating public and patient involvement in basic and preclinical health research. PLoS One. 2019;14(5):e0216600.

MacMillan C. Contracts and equality: the dangers of non-disclosure agreements in English law. Eur Rev Contract Law. 2022;18(2):127–58.

Mallonee S, Fowler C, Istre GR. Bridging the gap between research and practice: a continuing challenge. Inj Prev. 2006;12(6):357.

Merchant A, Rose G, Moody G, Matthews L. Effect of university heritage and reputation on attitudes of prospective students. Int J Nonprofit Volunt Sect Mark. 2014;20:20.

NIHR, CSOS, HCRW, PHA. UK standards for public involvement. 2018.. Available from: https://sites.google.com/nihr.ac.uk/pi-standards/home

Polk M. Achieving the promise of transdisciplinarity: a critical exploration of the relationship between transdisciplinary research and societal problem solving. Sustain Sci. 2014;9(4):439–51.

Reed MS. The research impact handbook. Kinnoir, Aberdeenshire: Fast Track Impact; 2016.

Richards DP, Cobey KD, Proulx L, Dawson S, de Wit M, Toupin-April K. Identifying potential barriers and solutions to patient partner compensation (payment) in research. Res Involv Engag. 2022;8(1):7.

Ryttberg M, Geschwind L. Organising professional support staff at higher education institutions: a multidimensional, continuous balancing act. Tert Educ Manag. 2021;27(1):47–58.

Saunders T. UKRI 2022.. 2024. Available from: https://www.ukri.org/blog/voices-how-public-engagement-improves-research-and-innovation/

Scivil. Scivil: the Flemish knowledge center for citizen science. Available from: https://www.scivil.be/en. n.d.

SFI. Science Foundation Ireland future innovator prize. SDG challenge 2024 call document. Dublin; 2024.

Shahid KT, McGee HY. The Academy's original sin: reflections on universities, slavery, and History's role in institutional reform. Ohio Valley History. 2021;21(2):92–110.

Szluka P, Csajbók E, Győrffy B. Relationship between bibliometric indicators and university ranking positions. Sci Rep. 2023;13(1):14193.

Tekic A, Willoughby KW. Configuring intellectual property management strategies in co-creation: a contextual perspective. Innovations. 2020;22(2):128–59.

Tekic A, Willoughby KW, Füller J. Different settings, different terms and conditions: the impact of intellectual property arrangements on co-creation project performance. J Prod Innov Manag. 2023;40(5):679–704.

UKRI. About the REF 2024a. Available from: https://ref.ac.uk/2014/about/background/

UKRI. Knowledge exchange framework UK 2024b.. Updated 5 August 2024. Available from: https://www.ukri.org/what-we-do/supporting-collaboration/supporting-collaboration-research-england/knowledge-exchange-framework/

UNICEF. Minimum quality standards and indicators for community engagement. New York; 2020.

Wellcome Trust. Using an engaged research approach 2024. Available from: https://wellcome.org/grant-funding/guidance/prepare-to-apply/using-engaged-research-approach.

WHO. WHO community engagement framework for quality, people-centred and resilient health services 2017. Available from: https://iris.who.int/bitstream/handle/10665/259280/WHO-HIS-SDS-2017.15-eng.pdf?sequence=1

Yep KS, Mitchell TD. Decolonizing community engagement: reimagining service learning through an ethnic studies lens. In: Dolgon C, Mitchell TD, Eatman TK, editors. The Cambridge handbook of service learning and community engagement. Cambridge handbooks in psychology. Cambridge: Cambridge University Press; 2017. p. 294–303.

Chapter 3
Engaged Research and Impact Case Studies

3.1 Introduction

Engaged research, characterised by collaborative efforts between researchers and community stakeholders, has gained prominence as a means to produce impactful, real-world solutions. This chapter delves into the essence of engaged research through a series of detailed case studies, highlighting the diverse methodologies and significant impacts that have emerged from such collaborations. By examining these examples in the area of social, health, and environmental impact, we can draw lessons and best practices for fostering a productive ecosystem for engaged research.

3.2 Social Impact Case Study

Correcting State Narratives on the Magdalene Laundries

3.2.1 Research Description

Magdalene Laundries were institutions where women and girls were forced to perform unpaid labour, such as laundry work, sewing, cleaning, and cooking, as a form of penance for violating moral codes. These establishments operated in Europe, North America, and Australia from the eighteenth to the twentieth centuries and were typically run by religious organisations.

An estimated 30,000 women were confined in Magdalene Laundries in Ireland during the two centuries in which they operated. However, the abuse and neglect endured by these women only began to come to light at the end of the twentieth

© The Author(s), under exclusive license to Springer Nature Switzerland AG 2024
E. R. Dorris et al., *Building the Ecosystem for Engaged Research*,
SpringerBriefs in Public Health, https://doi.org/10.1007/978-3-031-82080-9_3

century. One such institution, Donnybrook Magdalene Laundry (DML), opened in 1837 and closed in 1992 (Coen et al. 2023). Dr Claire McGettrick of Justice for Magdalenes Research, a collaborator on this project, has so far recorded the names of 315 women and girls who died there (McGettrick 2023).

In 2013, the Irish government published a report which outlined significant state collusion with the Magdalene Laundries (Ireland 2013). The report claimed that the laundries generally operated on a break-even basis without turning a profit, and that financial records for DML did not survive.

An interdisciplinary research team led by Dr Mark Coen and Professor Katherine O'Donnell of University College Dublin, along with Dr Maeve O'Rourke of University of Galway, has examined this institution in greater detail, asking two key research questions:

1. What can be learned about the Magdalene Laundry system as a whole by examining the operation, development, and legacy of one individual institution within that system?
2. To what extent can the story of a particular Magdalene Laundry be told without access to the institutional archives held by the religious congregation that managed it?

Inspiration for the research came when Dr Coen watched a YouTube video (2016) showing how well the institution and its artifacts were preserved.

From the outset, the team worked closely with survivors of DML to address these questions. Since 2011, Professor O'Donnell has led the collection of a substantial range of oral histories, which provided prompts as to what avenues the researchers might explore, and how they might interpret their findings. The team also arranged site visits with survivors, where their insights guided the researchers who were studying the architecture and archaeology of the laundry and piecing together a history of the institution from a diverse range of documentary sources.

Insights from survivors of DML were doubly important here, since the Religious Sisters of Charity, who owned and managed the laundry, refused to give the research team access to their archives. This prompted the team to explore every conceivable option to obtain information about the institution.

The researchers found that DML, and other institutions like it, were highly visible until 1970, mentioned in newspapers and in sermons broadcast on national radio. They also found that as early as 1903 a commentator wrote in a well-known book *Priests and People in Ireland* (McCarthy 1903) that DML was a prison-like institution where labour exploitation took place, and that in the 1940s the Department of Defence cancelled a contract for military laundry with DML because the nuns were not paying wages. These findings demonstrate that the labour practices of the laundries were regarded as suspect, at least in some quarters, far earlier than previously thought.

Contrary to Irish state narratives, the team found that financial records did in fact survive, and that DML was a profitable enterprise, recording healthy annual financial surpluses.

3.2.2 Research Impact Achieved

3.2.2.1 Academic Impact

The team's research methods were radically interdisciplinary: they analysed archaeological evidence from the DML site, architectural plans of demolished buildings, and grave markers in the institution's cemetery. They also discovered financial records and correspondence on the site of the abandoned institution. They consulted applications for planning permission; electoral registers; census data; death registers; wills and charitable bequests; government reports; death notices; obituaries and advertisements in magazines and newspapers; radio broadcasts; court cases; state departmental records; diocesan archives; books published by religious congregations; drawings in the Irish Architectural Archive; as well as memoirs, biographies, and survivor oral histories.

Their contribution to developing a methodology for writing institutional histories has been publicly acknowledged. Reviewing the researchers' book *A Dublin Magdalene Laundry: Donnybrook and Church-State Power in Ireland* in the *Irish Times*, Catriona Crowe, formerly of the National Archives, stated that the research "has created a template... for how to write an informative history of a religious order or a religious institution without recourse to the still closed records of these organisations, who ran a shadow state fully sanctioned by government".

3.2.2.2 Political Impact

Dr Coen, Professor O'Donnell, and the team located important financial records which demonstrate, in detail, that DML operated annually with a significant financial surplus, disproving the official state report. They also disproved the report's finding that there was no evidence to support a claim that DML was awarded a military contract in the 1940s. The team not only proved that such a contract was awarded but also that it was cancelled by the state because the nuns were in breach of a fair wages clause in their contract with the Department of Defence (Coen et al. 2023).

The project's oral histories and archaeological and architectural analysis of the buildings show how daily life and work was designed to be punitive, which further undermines the state's insistence that these were benign institutions where no physical or human rights abuses took place (O'Donnell et al. 2010).

Having published their findings, Dr Coen and Professor O'Donnell, along with Dr Maeve O'Rourke, have had constructive meetings with members of the Oireachtas, including the Tánaiste, where they discussed the urgent need for legislation to ensure that institutional archives are preserved and ultimately become accessible to the citizens of Ireland. Two members of the Irish parliament, Ivana Bacik TD and Marian Harkin TD, have quoted from the book in contributions in the Dáil on this subject (Ireland 2023).

3.2.2.3 Cultural and Social Impact

The financial records and correspondence that the team found on the laundry site are now being digitised and will be made available via the University of Galway archive. They have brokered agreements between the current owners of the DML site and the National Museum of Ireland (NMI) to successfully transfer artefacts—including laundry machinery and religious iconography from the derelict laundry—into the national collection. Discussions with survivors informed the curator from the NMI on what items to acquisition for the collection. The NMI regards this collection as central to its planned new museum on the site of the former Magdalene Laundry in Sean McDermott Street (Ireland 2023).

Survivors of institutional abuse attended the launch of the book. The team continues to work with survivors to ensure that Irish society—through publications, the development of teaching and learning materials, public exhibitions and lectures, and media interviews—better understands how class and gender politics have caused and continue to cause significant disadvantage in our society.

3.2.3 Important Insights for Engaged Research

3.2.3.1 Engagement with Survivors to Gather Testimonies

A key lesson from this case study is how researchers engaged with survivors to gather their testimonies by means of a funded research project. "Magdalene Institutions: Recording an Oral and Archival History" was a Government of Ireland Collaborative Research Project funded by the Irish Research Council which was led by Professor Katherine O'Donnell at University College Dublin.

The overall objective of the project was to contribute towards a better understanding of the Magdalene Laundry system that existed in Ireland through the gathering and study of testimonies from people who are directly or indirectly related to these institutions.

The Magdalene Oral History Project archive contains 84 transcripts (from 97 interviewees). The interviews and archival documents are available to the public through UCD Archives, the Irish Qualitative Data Archive, and the project website (JFMR 2013; O'Donnell et al. 2010).

The personal accounts and testimonies of survivors have been crucial in challenging the state's narrative and leading to the impacts described in this case study. These testimonies have highlighted the severe mistreatment, forced labour, and violations of human rights that occurred in the laundries.

The stories and testimonies of survivors have shifted public perception, leading to a greater understanding of the injustices committed in the Magdalene Laundries. This change in perception has been essential for garnering public support for the survivors' cause.

3.2.3.2 Engagement with Politicians

After publishing their findings, the researchers held productive meetings with members of the Irish Parliament, including the Tánaiste (Deputy Prime Minister). During these discussions, they emphasised the urgent need for legislation to preserve institutional archives and ensure they become accessible to the citizens of Ireland. Members of the Irish Parliament also cited the researchers work in parliamentary debates.

3.2.3.3 Engagement with Media

Engagement with the media played a crucial role in correcting state narratives on the Magdalene Laundries in Ireland by providing a platform for survivors and researchers to share their stories and findings with a wider audience. Media coverage helped to raise public awareness about the true nature of these institutions, highlighting the abuse and exploitation that occurred within them. This public exposure put pressure on the government to acknowledge past wrongdoings and reconsider the official narratives that downplayed or denied the extent of the maltreatment.

Journalists and media outlets investigated and reported on the discrepancies between state reports and the evidence uncovered by the researchers, further undermining the state's initial claims (Irish Times 2023; Spain 2023). The media also facilitated public discussions and debates, encouraging a national reckoning with this aspect of Ireland's history. Additionally, documentaries, news articles, and interviews with survivors provided powerful personal testimonies that resonated with the public and policymakers alike, fostering a greater understanding and empathy towards the victims and reinforcing the call for justice and transparency.

3.3 Environmental Impact Case Study

iSCAPE: Improving the Smart Control of Air Pollution in Europe

3.3.1 Research Description

Air pollution is one of society's greatest challenges, killing around seven million people every year. A total 400,000 of these premature deaths are in Europe. Every day, nine out of ten people breathe air with high levels of pollutants (WHO 2023). Air pollution also contributes to climate change and causes a range of environmental effects, like acid rain, ozone depletion, and damage to crops, forests, and wildlife. Addressing this challenge requires a concerted effort across society.

The iSCAPE project, coordinated by Professor Francesco Pilla, was a European research project that worked on advancing the control of air quality and carbon emissions in European cities. It tackled the problem by studying policy interventions, behaviour changes of citizens' lifestyles, and "Passive Control Systems" (PCSs)—things like trees, hedges, and coatings that can affect air pollution without using any power. Crucially, the project pioneered a co-design approach, developing solutions with a wide range of stakeholders using a so-called living lab framework. This means collaborating with citizens and decision-makers to develop and trial measures in real places. The work was carried out in six fully operating European cities, demonstrating the effectiveness of bottom-up approaches compared to more traditional top-down approaches to tackling pollution.

The team looked at different measures in each city:

- Bologna, Italy (trees and photocatalytic coating)
- Bottrop, Germany (urban design and planning)
- Dublin, Ireland (low-boundary walls)
- Guildford, UK (hedges)
- Hasselt, Belgium (behavioural interventions)
- Vantaa, Finland (green roofs and walls)

These studies were enhanced by scientific simulations to evaluate the measures at three different scales: the street, the neighbourhood, and the urban scale. iSCAPE also looked at how successful these measures would be in future climate scenarios, which enabled the team to develop air pollution control strategies that are effective in the short and the medium-long term.

This combination of approaches allowed Professor Pilla and colleagues to produce robust scientific results (over 50 peer-reviewed publications) and leverage the support of the wider community (over 100 citizens actively involved in producing the evidence) to influence policymakers to put the findings into practice.

3.3.2 Research Impact Achieved

3.3.2.1 Policy Impact

Local stakeholders—including decision-makers, environmental agencies, and city administrations—were directly involved in the process of producing guidelines for the measures developed through iSCAPE.

These guidelines include "Using Green Infrastructure to Protect People from Air Pollution", published by the Mayor of London, and "Implementing Green Infrastructure for Air Pollution Abatement: General Recommendations for Management and Plant Species Selection". The various guidelines fostered widespread adoption and application of nature-based solutions to tackle local air pollution challenges. iSCAPE also produced nine actionable policy briefs and promoted them through the World Health Organization (WHO) network, to facilitate the uptake of all the other key results of the project (iSCAPE 2019a, 2020).

3.3.2.2   Environmental Impact

Ultimately, these guidelines being adopted around Europe has had multiple benefits in terms of alleviating climate change impacts, increasing biodiversity, enhancing people's well-being, and increasing resilience to flooding and other risks. All the produced results and actionable policy briefs are freely available, ensuring further policies around the world will benefit from the research, and helping additional cities tackle air pollution and climate change (iSCAPE 2019a).

3.3.2.3   Social Impact

iSCAPE Living Labs brought together a great variety of urban stakeholders, including city representatives, researchers, businesses, and citizens, to solve complex city challenges around air pollution and climate change.

During the project, iSCAPE Living Labs delivered numerous engagement activities, increasing citizen awareness and knowledge of air pollution, its impacts, and how to address it. The events involved a wide range of activities, from creating pop-up green spaces as part of the "wandering trees" initiative in Bottrop, to citizen science workshops with low-cost sensors in all the six Living Labs.

One such activity took place in a school, where children co-developed passive control systems for air pollution using LEGO bricks (Getz et al. 2018). This has since been formalised in a framework which will be replicated by the International Red Cross in schools in over 50 countries in Eurasia.

3.3.2.4   Technological Impact

iSCAPE developed two low-cost sensors to facilitate these activities: a citizen science sensor (Smart Citizen Kits) for grassroots activities with local communities aimed at raising awareness of air pollution, and a more advanced monitoring station to assess the impacts of the piloted interventions. The team developed an online guide to facilitate wider use of the Smart Citizen Kits (iSCAPE 2019b).

3.3.2.5   Academic Impact

iSCAPE produced several impactful results, advancing the state of the art and significantly contributing to scientific knowledge about the effectiveness of nature-based solutions and behavioural change initiatives to tackle air pollution and related climate change issues. More than 50 publications have arisen from the project.

A sustainability plan for extending the lifespan and impact of the project was developed to ensure that the Living Lab components—including physical and virtual infrastructure, knowledge, and skills—are sustained beyond the project and continue contributing to local urban innovation activities (Schaaf 2019).

3.3.3   Important Insights for Engaged Research

Overall, the iSCAPE project highlights the effectiveness of an engaged research approach that integrates stakeholder collaboration, innovative technologies, and evidence-based policy interventions to address complex societal challenges like air pollution.

3.3.3.1   Stakeholder Engagement

iSCAPE emphasised the importance of involving a wide range of stakeholders, including citizens, environmental agencies, and policymakers, in co-designing solutions to air pollution. This collaborative approach ensured that the interventions were practical, acceptable, and tailored to local needs.

By involving citizens directly in research activities, iSCAPE raised public awareness about air pollution and its impacts. This engagement helped build community support for air quality initiatives and fostered a sense of ownership and responsibility among the participants.

3.3.3.2   Use of Technology to Engage Citizens

iSCAPE developed low-cost air quality sensors that empowered local communities to monitor air pollution. This technological advancement not only provided valuable data but also raised awareness and engaged citizens in pollution control efforts.

3.3.3.3   Evidence-Based Policy Interventions

The findings from iSCAPE informed various policy interventions, showcasing the project's ability to bridge the gap between research and practical policy implementation. This alignment with policy frameworks was crucial for scaling and sustaining the project's impact.

3.4 Health Impact Case Study

#WeAreNotWaiting: Tackling Diabetes Through Patient-led Research and Open-Source Innovation

3.4.1 Research Description

Managing diabetes is a continuous, around-the-clock responsibility. In addition to life-threatening physical complications, the burden of diabetes can lead to psychological distress, anxiety, and depression for people with diabetes and their families.

The concept of an automated insulin delivery (AID) system (software that automatically adjusts insulin dosage with a pump according to predicted blood sugar levels) is a promising approach to managing diabetes (Braune et al. 2022). It improves glucose levels while reducing the emotional and cognitive burden of living with diabetes. An algorithm takes over decision-making from the user, calculating predicted glucose levels every 5 min and adjusting insulin delivery accordingly—similarly to the pancreas of a person without diabetes.

However, the research, commercial development, and regulatory approval of such technologies have been fragmented and slow. As a result, tech-savvy patients initiated the grassroots movement "#WeAreNotWaiting" and developed their own AID systems (Braune et al. 2021). Based on the principles of open-source sharing, this online community has helped over 10,000 people worldwide to build their own system for automated insulin delivery, and the uptake continues to grow.

Until recently, evidence on the safety and effectiveness of these systems has been lacking, as has evidence on the lived experiences of people using them. To address this gap, an international team of interdisciplinary researchers co-founded the OPEN project in 2019, with the aim of examining the outcomes experienced by users of open-source AID, and the implications for more widespread use among people with diabetes (O'Donnell et al. 2019).

The team found significant improvements across all participants (in terms of self-reported clinical outcomes), regardless of age and gender. The most significant transformation was in relation to quality of life. There was almost universal consensus among participants that these systems were life-changing and brought with them improvements in sleep quality that had been previously unimaginable (Braune et al. 2019). This is highlighted by a parent of a 12-year-old boy from the United Kingdom, who was three when diagnosed: "If I could give my pancreas to my son, I would. This is the next best available option".

However, participants also highlighted the multiple challenges of building AID systems (O'Donnell et al. 2023). Major barriers include sourcing the necessary components, lack of confidence in one's own technological knowledge and skills, perceived time and energy required to build a system, and fear of losing support from healthcare providers. The support of the wider diabetes community was seen as crucial for overcoming some of these hurdles.

3.4.2 Research Impact Achieved

3.4.2.1 Political and Technological Impact

The OPEN project is establishing a scientific evidence base around open-source AID. It is helping patients, healthcare professionals, researchers, industry, and regulators to recognise the value and importance of user-led, open-source innovation and the real-world evidence emerging from it (O'Donnell et al. 2019).

In 2020, OPEN teamed up with 48 medical experts and 4 legal experts across 25 countries to create a consensus statement on the safe and ethical use of these systems, which currently have no regulatory approval in clinical practice (Braune et al. 2022). The consensus statement, which has been endorsed by several international professional diabetes organisations—including the International Diabetes Federation and International Society for Pediatric and Adolescent Diabetes—is published in *The Lancet Diabetes & Endocrinology*.

This is the first time that international guidance on open-source AID has been provided to healthcare professionals. The guidelines will be particularly important in providing education and reassurance to healthcare providers who are increasingly encountering these systems in their clinical practice. Alongside other guidance that will likely emerge in the future, it is expected to help policymakers deal with the legal and regulatory dilemmas that open-source innovation presents to formal healthcare systems.

3.4.2.2 Health Impact

Around the world, there are roughly 10,000 people using an open-source AID. However, based on membership of DIY social media groups, the team estimates that the number of people interested in building one of these systems is several times that figure.

Through the work of OPEN, those interested in DIY solutions can make an informed decision about whether an open-source AID system would help them to manage their diabetes. As a result, uptake will likely increase, improving patients' clinical outcomes and their quality of life. Research by the OPEN team also provides evidence of the impact of growing inequalities in access to these life-enhancing technologies, supporting the work of those advocating for increased affordability and access for all (O'Donnell et al. 2023).

3.4.2.3   Social Impact

Importantly, OPEN has also sparked significant interest within the diabetes community and the wider public. For example, a public engagement event aimed at promoting awareness of the initial findings of the OPEN project held at UCD in May 2019 attracted over 150 people, including healthcare professionals, medical device manufacturers, and people living with diabetes. Similar public engagement events have been staged in Copenhagen and Barcelona. This continued during COVID-19 when the OPEN team presented at the Loop and Learn session, a regular online workshop for people with diabetes who want to learn more about open-source AID systems.

3.4.2.4   Academic Impact

The team has published open-access articles in several prestigious journals on clinical outcomes of people using these systems, as well as their motivations for building them. Two senior researchers from the OPEN team are currently guest-editing a special issue of Diabetic Medicine on user-led diabetes technology.

OPEN has gained recognition for its uniquely user-centred and patient-driven approach, both within the scientific community and beyond. For example, in 2020 it was awarded the Berlin Institute for Health QUEST Patient and Stakeholder Engagement Award, and in 2021 the BIH QUEST Patient & Stakeholder Engagement Grant for a follow-up project that facilitates direct patient engagement in academic teaching of future doctors, clinical researchers, and healthcare providers.

3.4.3   Important Insights for Engaged Research

This case study highlights several key takeaways for engaged researchers.

3.4.3.1   Empowerment Through Collaboration

The initiative showcases the importance of empowering patients to take control of their health through collaboration. By engaging directly with patients, researchers can better understand the real-world challenges and needs, leading to more relevant and impactful research outcomes. This collaboration not only benefits the patients but also enhances the research process by incorporating diverse perspectives and expertise.

3.4.3.2   Open-Source Technologies

The use of open-source platforms and tools in the #WeAreNotWaiting movement illustrates the potential of open innovation to drive rapid advancements in healthcare. By sharing data, software, and findings openly, researchers and patients can co-create solutions that are immediately accessible and adaptable, fostering a community-driven approach to problem-solving.

3.4.3.3   Patient-Led Advocacy and Research

The case study underscores the significant role that patient advocacy can play in advancing research and innovation. Patients involved in the #WeAreNotWaiting movement were not just passive subjects but active researchers and developers, highlighting the shift towards more inclusive and participatory research methodologies.

3.4.3.4   Barriers and Enablers

The case study identifies systemic barriers, such as regulatory challenges and the need for validation and standardisation, which can hinder the progress of patient-led initiatives. Engaging with regulators early in the project lifecycle is recommended as a result.

However, the case study also highlights enablers like community support, technological advancements, and open-source platforms that facilitate the success of such movements. By integrating these insights, engaged researchers can foster a more inclusive and impactful research environment, leveraging the strengths and contributions of all stakeholders involved.

3.5   Summary and Key Messages

Engaged research holds great potential for generating meaningful impacts by aligning academic enquiry with community needs. By fostering strong partnerships, respecting local knowledge, and addressing systemic enablers and barriers, engaged research can drive significant positive change across various disciplines. The case studies presented in this chapter illustrate the diverse ways in which engaged research can be applied. These real-life examples highlight how a cultivation of a robust environment that supports and sustains engaged research can lead to lasting and meaningful societal impact.

Key Messages

1. Foster collaborative networks by establishing partnerships between universities, community organisations, and policymakers to create a supportive infrastructure for engaged research.
2. Support capacity building by providing training and resources for researchers and community members to develop skills necessary for effective collaboration.
3. Advocate for funding models that prioritise long-term, community-driven research projects.
4. Promote policy integration by actively encouraging the incorporation of research findings into policy and practice to amplify impact.

References

Anonymous. Abandoned Magdalene laundry in Donnybrook, Dublin, Ireland. YouTube2016. (n.d.) https://www.youtube.com/watch?v=YETH7W0yCBg

Braune K, O'Donnell S, Cleal B, Lewis D, Tappe A, Willaing I, et al. Real-world use of Do-it-yourself artificial pancreas Systems in Children and Adolescents with Type 1 diabetes: online survey and analysis of self-reported clinical outcomes. JMIR Mhealth Uhealth. 2019;7(7):e14087.

Braune K, Gajewska KA, Thieffry A, Lewis DM, Froment T, O'Donnell S, et al. Why #WeAreNotWaiting—motivations and self-reported outcomes among users of open-source automated insulin delivery systems: multinational survey. J Med Internet Res. 2021;23(6):e25409.

Braune K, Lal RA, Petruželková L, Scheiner G, Winterdijk P, Schmidt S, et al. Open-source automated insulin delivery: international consensus statement and practical guidance for healthcare professionals. Lancet Diabetes Endocrinol. 2022;10(1):58–74.

Coen M, O'Donnell K, O'Rourke M. A Dublin Magdalene laundry: donnybrook and church-state power in Ireland. London: Bloomsbury Academic; 2023.

Getz I, Evitts S, Pilla F, Stibe S. The air we breathe: eBook; 2018.

Ireland, Government of Report of the inter-departmental committee to establish the facts of state involvement with the Magdalen laundries. In: Justice Do, editor. Dublin: Government of Ireland; 2013.

Ireland, Government of Church-State Relations Dáil Éireann Debate, Wednesday - 22 March 2023. In: Oireachtas Hot, editor 2023.

Ireland, Government of Dáil Éireann debate -Wednesday, 8 Mar 2023.

Ireland, Government of National Centre—Background and current status. In: Department of Children E, Disability, Integration and Youth editor. Dublin. 2023.

Irish Times T. A Magdalene laundry and its clients: Holles street, Fitzwilliam tennis Club, Captain Americas Irish Times 2023 4 March 2023.

iSCAPE. iSCAPE Scientific and other reports. 2019a.

iSCAPE. Smart Citizen Kit and guides 2019b. Available from: https://docs.smartcitizen. me/#open-source

iSCAPE. Smart Control of Air Pollution—Policy Briefs series 2020. Available from: https://www. iscapeproject.eu/policy-briefs/

Justice for Magdalenes Research [Internet]. 2013. [cited 2024]. Available from: http://jfmresearch. com/home/oralhistoryproject/.

McCarthy M. Priests and people in Ireland. Dublin: Hodges Figgis; 1903.

McGettrick C. Guerrilla archive: donnybrook and the Magdalene names project. In: Coen MOD, Katherine; O'Rourke, Maeve, editor. A Dublin Magdalene laundry: donnybrook and church-state power in Ireland. London: Bloomsbury Academic; 2023.

O'Donnell K, Pembroke S, McGettrick C. Magdalene Oral history collection: Irish qualitative data archive; 2010.

O'Donnell S, Lewis D, Marchante Fernández M, Wäldchen M, Cleal B, Skinner T, et al. Evidence on user-led innovation in diabetes technology (the OPEN project): protocol for a mixed methods study. JMIR Res Protoc. 2019;8(11):e15368.

O'Donnell S, Cooper D, Chen Y, Ballhausen H, Lewis DM, Froment T, et al. Barriers to uptake of open-source automated insulin delivery systems: analysis of socioeconomic factors and perceived challenges of adults with type 1 diabetes from the OPEN survey. Diabetes Res Clin Pract. 2023;197:110235.

Schaaf K. Citizen science guide. In: An actionable guide for living labs; 2019. Available from: https://www.iscapeproject.eu/wp-content/uploads/2019/09/iSCAPE-CitizenScience-Guide.pdf.

Spain S. Fine or jail time needed for mishandling of Magdalene laundries documents. RTE. 2023. 10 Mar 2023.

WHO. WHO ambient air quality database, 2022 update: status report. World Health Organization; 2023.

Chapter 4
What's Next for Engaged Research?

4.1 Introduction

The research and development landscape is undergoing rapid change. Policies and future trends in research indicate we may be on a brink of a new era in research. In addition to digital technologies, as global challenges become more complex, multi-stakeholder partnerships between universities, industry, government, and other organisations are being increasingly recognised as essential for advancing knowledge and translating breakthroughs into real-world applications. At the same time, research performing higher education institutions (HEIs) and other publicly funded research performing organisations (RPOs) are facing new challenges from the shifting political landscapes, declines in public trust, and the challenges in leadership as the goals and expectations of publicly funded research and innovation becomes increasingly more complex (Clark et al. 2024).

Engaged research has come a long way in a relatively short period. It has moved from the periphery of academic practice to a more central role in many research performing organisations. This shift has been driven by various factors, including the increasing recognition of the value of diverse perspectives in research, the demand for research that has a tangible impact on society, and the growing expectations for accountability and transparency in the use of public funds. However, as engaged research becomes more mainstream, it also faces new challenges. These include issues related to the scalability of engagement practices, the need for robust and flexible infrastructure, robust processes, increased support capacity at RPOs, effective policy, and sustainable funding mechanisms. To address these challenges, it is essential to look ahead and consider what steps can be taken to ensure that engaged research not only survives but also thrives in the future.

© The Author(s), under exclusive license to Springer Nature Switzerland AG 2024
E. R. Dorris et al., *Building the Ecosystem for Engaged Research*,
SpringerBriefs in Public Health, https://doi.org/10.1007/978-3-031-82080-9_4

4.2   From Playing Catch-up to Sustainable Growth in an Expanding Area

Engaged research is growing rapidly. Between 2014 and 2023, there were 83,507 academic publications globally related to engaged research (Fig. 4.1; see Appendix for methods used). There is continued year-on-year growth in the volume of publications. The number of total publications nearly tripled during this 10-year period. The breakdown of research disciplines represented in the dataset can be found in Fig. 4.2. Traditionally, engaged research has been primarily associated with the medical and social science fields (see Chap. 1), and indeed these disciplines contributed to half of the total research outputs. However, what is particularly interesting is the trends in growth from 2014 to 2023 across less traditionally engaged disciplines (see Fig. 4.3). Engaged research in environmental, agricultural, and biological sciences has seen a fivefold increase across this time period, demonstrating a significant shift as other disciplines increasingly adopt engaged research methodologies. This trend is not due to change in the short term (Jah 2024).

Engaged research is part of a wider democratic movement to involve citizens in making the decisions that affect them and their communities. The policy drivers behind the growth of engaged research are not only research policies but also wider accountability and competitiveness policies. The rise in the deliberative democracy model for decision-making has greatly influenced the research realm, especially in the European Union (EU; Fiorino 1990). The deliberative model, where publics are actively involved in decision-making processes, acknowledges that uncertainty exists as evidence is incomplete (Fig. 4.4). Deliberative democracy recognises that the framing and judgement involved in assessing incomplete bodies of evidence are not solely dictated by scientific reasoning and acknowledges that citizens and

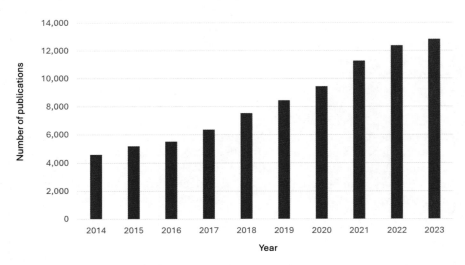

Fig. 4.1 Number of research publications linked to engaged research per year

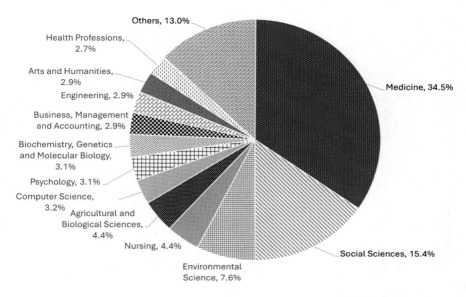

Fig. 4.2 Percentage of research publications linked to engaged research per discipline from 2014 to 2023

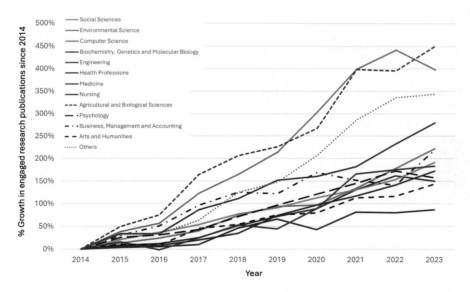

Fig. 4.3 Research discipline growth trends of research publications linked to engaged research since 2014

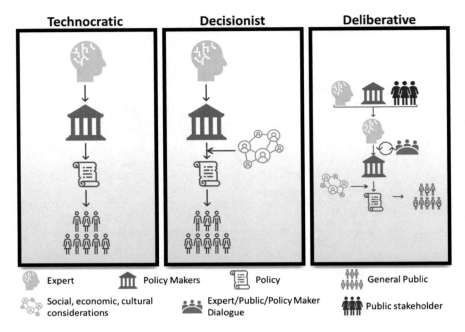

Fig. 4.4 The evolution of decision-making models in policy has influenced engaged research. Traditional policy models had an expert-led approach (technocratic model). In the late 1990s, in Western Europe, there was a move towards acknowledging public views and beliefs are both legitimate and necessary for informed decision-making on policy (decisionist model). More recently, there has been movement towards involving citizens not just in debating policy options but also in creating the policy themselves (deliberative model)

communities can bring value and knowledge to policy development (Stirling 2003). This reflects the underlying concept of engaged research, and the upwards trend in engaged research can be seen as a form of civic participation that strengthens democratic processes. In summary, the growth in engaged research is evident in both research outputs and underlying policy trends. Engaged research approaches are not going away and now is the time to focus on building the ecosystem we want and need instead of trying to force it to fit into a mould that doesn't work.

4.2.1   Research Movements Important for the Future of Engaged Research

In many countries, public funds are a primary source of research funding (Gibbons and NCSES 2022; UIS 2024). There is an increasing demand for transparency and public accountability in the use of public funds, including those used for research. Engaged research may help to demonstrate that the research is relevant and beneficial to society. It acknowledges that knowledge produced by publicly funded research is a public good, and researchers and RPOs have a responsibility to maximise its impact. Responsible research and innovation (RRI) is the term for integrating approaches within research to align both the research process and its outcomes with the values, needs, and expectations of society (European Commission 2012). The RRI framework was adopted by the European Commission in the early 2010s. The goal is to improve research integrity by fostering the design of inclusive and sustainable research and innovation. RRI is an aspect of the science with and for society movement, and it encompasses public engagement (including engaged research), open access, gender, ethics, science education, governance, and the promotion of institutional change to accommodate these (Owen et al. 2012).

RRI is aligned with the principles of open science (Shelley-Egan et al. 2020). Open science refers to the movement towards making scientific research, data, and dissemination accessible to all levels of society, ranging from professional researchers to the general public. This approach advocates for transparency in the research process, the sharing of methodologies and data, and the free availability of research outputs. By dismantling barriers to knowledge and fostering collaborative environments, open science aims to democratise the scientific enterprise, enhance reproducibility, and accelerate innovation. The future potential benefits of open science are manifold, including increased public trust in science, the broadening of participation in research from underrepresented groups, and the potential for more rapid and equitable societal advancements (Song et al. 2022). As the scientific community increasingly embraces open science practices, the potential for transformative impacts on both research quality and societal well-being becomes more pronounced, ultimately fostering a more inclusive and innovative global research ecosystem.

The European Commission identified eight pillars to promote open science (European Commission 2018a). Pillar five is citizen science, defined as the voluntary participation of non-professional scientists in research and innovation at different stages and at different levels of engagement, from shaping research agendas and policies to gathering, processing, and analysing data, as well as assessing the outcomes of research. The European Research Area (ERA) policy agenda includes the promotion of open science as one of its key priorities (European Commission 2022a, b). The ERA roadmap supports member states in adopting policies that foster open science practices and emphasises the need for systematic monitoring of open science policies, with specific indicators and benchmarks to assess progress at both national and EU levels. Horizon Europe (2021–2027), the EU's primary funding programme for research and innovation, requires citizen engagement across all of its missions. The National Institutes of Health (NIH) in the United States also requires evidence of citizen engagement in the research process.

The establishment of a European Science for Policy (S4P) ecosystem aims to create coherent S4P approaches, enhance knowledge sharing, and promote best practices across Europe (Pedersen and Krieger 2023). This ecosystem will support the development of higher-quality policies, enhance competitiveness, and strengthen Europe's Open Strategic Autonomy through closer collaboration and mutual learning among EU Member States and associated countries. In this ecosystem, researchers, advisors, knowledge brokers, and policymakers will collaborate to generate relevant scientific knowledge and produce actionable policy options based on the best available science. This collaboration will help bridge the gap between scientists and policymakers, fostering trust and acceptance among societal and political actors, and improving the success rate of policy implementation. The European S4P ecosystem will also encourage the growth and interconnection of S4P ecosystems across Europe by promoting knowledge sharing, building competencies, offering alternative career paths, and recognising researchers and advisors engaged in policymaking. It will be based on commonly accepted research ethics and high levels of integrity, enhancing the quality and societal value of scientific evidence used in policymaking and strengthening democratic processes. The ecosystem is expected to build trust at multiple levels: among S4P actors (scientists, advisors, and policymakers) through collaborative efforts and independence, and among citizens, fostering confidence in both science and governance. Engaging citizens and diverse societal actors in the S4P ecosystem will highlight the role of scientific insights in policy design and implementation, thereby reinforcing democratic processes and improving societal outcomes.

In the United States, several key policies and legislative frameworks promote open science, with specific emphasis on public or citizen engagement in the research process. Executive Orders on Open Government and Transparency have emphasised open government principles, including transparency, participation, and collaboration (White House 2024). These orders fostered open science by promoting the availability and accessibility of government-held information, including research data. This laid the groundwork for public engagement in science by encouraging federal agencies to involve citizens in the development and implementation of policies, research agendas, and data-sharing initiatives. The Federal Crowdsourcing and Citizen Science Act (2016) encourages public participation in scientific research by allowing citizens to contribute to data collection, analysis, and problem-solving efforts (USA 2016). This policy formalises the role of citizen science in federal research, fostering greater public involvement in scientific enquiry and innovation. The Office of Science and Technology Policy (OSTP) Memo on Open Science both accelerates the dissemination of scientific knowledge to the public and emphasises the importance of engaging the public in the research process, encouraging greater transparency and accountability in federally funded research (Nelson and OSTP 2022). The recognition of crowdsourcing and that engaging citizens can foster innovation is particularly relevant in sectors like technology and environmental research, where public insights can drive market-oriented innovations.

Engagement in environmental research has also been driven by the UN's Sustainable Development Goals (SDGs). The SDGs emphasise the need for inclusive and participatory decision-making (UN 2015). Research related to sustainability challenges often includes engagement to ensure that local knowledge and perspectives inform solutions. Additionally, climate action policies and the just transition to net zero often emphasise the importance of involving and protecting vulnerable populations who may be disproportionately affected by climate change and the transition to a low-carbon economy. Policies such as the new European

Bauhaus, the policy and funding initiative of the European Commission (2021) focused on the built environment and lifestyles under the green transition, also have a significant focus on social inclusion. The establishment of climate-related citizen assemblies (UK 2019; Germany 2019; Spain 2022), national dialogues (Ireland 2021, 2024), and multi-stakeholder advisory boards (Canada 2021) for citizen engagement in climate policy reflects the growing uptake of engaged research in climate-related disciplines (Elstub et al. 2021; Citizen Initiative on Climate 2021; MITECO 2022; Ireland 2021, 2024; and Canada 2021). Ensuring that affected communities are engaged and their needs addressed is crucial for achieving just and inclusive climate action.

Policies focused on equity and inclusion often push for citizen engagement in research to ensure that marginalised voices are heard and that research outcomes benefit all segments of society. These policies focus on research that is participatory, equitable, and reflective of diverse perspectives. Policies that mandate or strongly encourage community-based participatory research (CBPR), where citizens, especially marginalised groups, are actively involved in research to address local issues (see Chap. 1), are often related to public health. In the United States, the National Institute on Minority Health and Health Disparities (NIMHD) has programmes that specifically fund research projects that involve CBPR approaches to address health disparities in minority communities (NIH 2024). These grants require that community partners are involved in all stages of the research, from planning and implementation to analysis and dissemination. The Centers for Disease Control and Prevention (CDC) Prevention Research Centers (PRCs) programme mandates that academic centres establish long-term partnerships with community stakeholders, ensuring that the research is community driven and directly addresses local public health needs (USA 2021). The UK government's public body that directs research and innovation funding, UK Research and Innovation (UKRI), has a commitment to both equality, diversity, and inclusion and public involvement across their portfolio (UKRI 2023). Through the previously mentioned RRI framework and programmes such as the European Social Fund Community-Led Local Development, there is a strong commitment within Europe to foster research and research adjacent policies that are socially relevant and inclusive (European Commission 2022a, b).

The value of research depends on how effectively the results are used. However, research impact assessment is complex, involving both political and socio-economic factors (MacDonogh et al. 2022). With the establishment of the European Research Area in 2020, a key objective was to improve research assessment and collaboration in Europe (DGRI 2022; European Commission 2020). Knowledge valorisation in the EU is a key policy objective that seeks to transform research outputs into tangible societal, economic, and environmental impacts. Valorisation is part of the wider strategy to enhance the competitiveness of Europe (European Commission 2024). The underlying thesis is that translation of knowledge generated in the EU into market-ready products, services, and policies can help the EU maintain its position as a global leader in innovation. Furthermore, knowledge valorisation promotes the sharing and use of research across borders and sectors, thereby supporting the development of a cohesive European Research Area (ERA), reinforcing collaboration between academia, industry, policymakers, and citizens. This approach ensures that the benefits of publicly funded research are maximised, aligning with the EU's broader goals of social cohesion, economic resilience, and sustainability.

The EU is focusing on citizen engagement in knowledge valorisation and has a code of practice and recommendations on how to promote and capture evidence of citizen engagement of knowledge valorisation (European Commission 2024). This frequently aligns with the vision and strategies of RPOs. Both the EU and RPOs want greater uptake of research and innovation results to foster economic and societal prosperity. The focus on citizen engagement is a recognition that involving the public in the research and innovation process can lead to more impactful, inclusive, and sustainable outcomes. The reasons underlying why the EU has a specific focus on knowledge valorisation through citizen engagement (or engaged research) include:

- Enhancing Societal Relevance: Citizen engagement ensures that research and innovation address the real needs and concerns of society. By involving citizens, the EU can better align outputs with societal priorities making research more relevant and responsive to the public.
- Promoting Trust and Transparency: When the public is actively involved in the research process, they are more likely to understand and accept the outcomes. This may reduce resistance to new technologies and policies.
- Driving Innovation: Involving end-users early in the innovation process encourages co-creation and user-centred design. More diverse voices can lead to valuable insights, experiences, and ideas that complement the expertise of researchers and innovators.
- Fostering Inclusivity and Equity: Including diverse perspectives, particularly from underrepresented or vulnerable communities, can reduce inequalities and make innovation more inclusive, reflecting the needs of all citizens. It can help to ensure that the benefits of knowledge valorisation are shared more equitably across different communities.
- Maximising Impact and Uptake: Engagement throughout the research cycle can help the results of knowledge valorisation be more widely accepted and adopted. This may lead to more efficient dissemination of innovations. Communities who feel a sense of ownership are more likely to support and advocate for the implementation of research outcomes.

The EU knowledge valorisation policy also includes a focus on efficient intellectual assets management. It recognises that good IP and asset management is needed to improve the chances of knowledge reaching the market and benefiting society (European Commission 2021). The Code of Practice on the Management of Intellectual Assets for Knowledge Valorisation promotes a harmonised, strategic, and responsible approach to managing intellectual assets (European Commission 2023). Its goal is to ensure that research outputs are translated into societal and economic benefits in line with the goals of the European Research Area. The Code promotes collaborative research by recommending processes should be implemented to facilitate IP sharing between organisations. It also supports the responsible transfer of knowledge and IP responsibly to industry and society. The code actively supports the development of specialised IP management skills to enhance university RPOs ability to achieve this. This again demonstrates the need for a comprehensive systems approach for sustainable embedding of engaged research and increased societal benefit.

Sustainable funding is required to support an engaged research ecosystem. Given the potential benefits of engaged research and its frequent alignment with strategic objectives and goals of research performing universities, the core funding for engaged research should arguably be jointly via government funding for research and development programmes in the higher education sector and investment from the Higher Education Institutions (HEIs) themselves. The current ecosystem is sub-optimal with challenges including the highly fragmented research landscape with widely varying levels of acknowledge, support, reward and recognition of the complexity, variety, and potential for engaged research to maximise societal benefits from research. There is a lack of overall coherence of the funding landscape. Engaged research is being adopted rapidly, albeit at different paces depending on discipline (see Fig. 4.3). Without more specific and dedicated long-term sustainable investment this growth cannot reap the intended long-term benefits. The lack of financial stability and permanence in infrastructure and personnel to support engaged research and the dependence on good will of societal partners is a real risk to the development of a mature ecosystem. Sustainability cannot be an individual organisation's task. It is reliant on sector-wide and system-wide changes. These changes are being referenced more frequently in policies, but the translation into real-world action, particularly in relation to core funding, is slow. For policies to turn into actions the need of dedicated core funding is key, otherwise systems cannot change.

4.2.2   Impact Evaluation and Engaged Research

Evaluating the impact of engaged research is critical for demonstrating its value to funders, policymakers, and the public. However, traditional metrics of academic success, such as publications and citations, are often inadequate for capturing the full range of impacts that engaged research can have (Reed 2018). Therefore, it is essential to develop new tools and frameworks for evaluating impact, which may include qualitative assessments, case studies, and participatory evaluation methods. A discussion of monitoring and evaluation at institutional level can be found in Chap. 2.

Some countries, such as the United Kingdom, have national level assessments and dedicated resources for evidencing research impact. For RPOs in other countries or regions with less dedicated funding and incentives, it can be difficult to know where to start. However, in order to build the knowledge base for engaged research it is undeniably important to collect evidence of impact. Documenting the impact of research involves a variety of methods and approaches, each suited to capturing different types of impact. A combination of these methods provides a more comprehensive understanding of the impact of research, catering to the various needs and expectations of the multiple research stakeholders. Table 4.1 lists

Table 4.1 Methods and approaches to capturing research impact

1. Quantitative metrics
Bibliometrics: Measures such as citation counts, h-index, and journal impact factors
Altmetrics: Metrics that capture attention in online environments, such as mentions on social media, news outlets, policy documents, and other online platforms
Grant and funding data: Amount and sources of research funding as indicators of the perceived value and potential impact
Patent citations: Number of patents citing the research as a measure of innovation and practical application
2. Qualitative methods
Case studies: Detailed descriptions of how research has influenced policy, practice, or further research
Narratives and testimonials: Personal accounts and stories from stakeholders, beneficiaries, or collaborators
Surveys and interviews: Direct feedback from researchers, practitioners, and other stakeholders about the impact of the research
3. Mixed methods
Logic models and theory of change: Frameworks that map out the pathways through which research is expected to lead to specific impacts
Impact narratives: Combining quantitative data with qualitative stories to provide a comprehensive picture of impact
Evaluation frameworks: Using a combination of methods to systematically assess research impact according to predefined criteria
4. Public engagement and media analysis
Media analysis: Monitoring and analysing media coverage of the research **Public engagement activities:** Evaluating the reach and effectiveness of public lectures, exhibitions, and other outreach activities
5. Policy analysis
Policy citations: Tracking references to research in policy documents and legislative texts **Policy changes:** Documenting instances where research has directly influenced policy decisions or practice guidelines
6. Economic analysis
Cost-benefit analysis: Assessing the economic impact of research, including cost savings or additional revenue generated **Economic impact studies:** Comprehensive studies to evaluate the broader economic effects of research, such as job creation and industry growth
7. Health and social impact
Health outcomes: Measuring changes in health outcomes that can be attributed to research **Social impact:** Assessing changes in social conditions, quality of life, or community well-being resulting from research
8. Academic and educational impact
Curriculum development: Influence on educational content and training programmes **Research training:** Impact on the development of researchers and their career progression

the many methods and approaches to capturing research impact. Which approaches are used will depend on the context of the research, its evaluation, and stakeholders. Often, a mix of qualitative, quantitative, and testimonial evidence is used to create a narrative presentation of the impacts of research. Case studies (see Chap. 3) are often used as a particularly valuable method for capturing the impact of research. They typically incorporate many of the methods mentioned in Table 4.1 into one narrative document.

Example: University College Dublin's Annual Research Impact Case Study Competition

The competition showcases the diverse ways research at UCD contributes to national and international advancements. Researchers from all disciplines across the university are invited to participate. Additionally, an "Engaged Research Impact Prize" is awarded to the finalist whose case study best represents the principles of engaged research. Researchers are supported via online resources and research impact workshops. The competition element incentivises researchers, encouraging and helping them to understand how to capture their impact and action actually doing so.

The key criteria for the competition's assessment rubric can be found in Fig. 4.5. Judges are both internal and external to the university, and often include research stakeholders such as policy actors, funders, and members of aligned public authorities. Thus, not only does this initiative drive the impact strategy agenda at the university, but it also acts as knowledge transfer of the breadth and impact of the universities research impact to key stakeholders in the research sector.

Horizon Europe is the European Union's primary funding mechanism for research and innovation from 2021 to 2027. The EU has developed a comprehensive framework to measure and assess the impact of engaged research at an overall programme level (European Commission 2018b). The monitoring and evaluation framework for this programme consists of three core components:

1. Annual performance monitoring: This involves tracking performance indicators over short-, medium-, and long-term periods along "key impact pathways" aligned with the programme's objectives. The use of targets and baselines is recommended where available.
2. Ongoing collection of data on programme management and programme implementation.
3. Two comprehensive evaluations: These (meta)-evaluations are conducted at the programme's mid-term and after its completion (ex-post).

The monitoring of the programme's performance is structured around impact pathways and their associated key indicators (Fig. 4.6). The objectives of Horizon Europe are categorised into three complementary impact areas, each tracked through

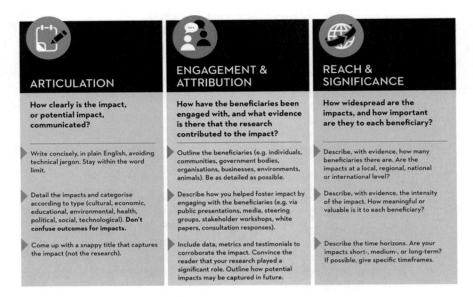

Fig. 4.5 The judging criteria for the Impact Case Study Competition and Engaged Research Impact prize. Judging is based on how clearly the impact has been articulated, the level of engagement with the people affected by the research, evidence that the research led to the impact, and the reach and significance of the impact to those who benefited from it

multiple pathways, highlighting the complex and non-linear nature of research and innovation (R&I) investments:

- Scientific impact: Focuses on fostering the creation and dissemination of "high-quality knowledge, skills, technologies, and solutions" (European Commission 2018c) to address global challenges.
- Societal impact: Aims to enhance the contribution "of research and innovation to developing, supporting, and implementing EU policies" (ibid), and to encourage the "adoption of innovative solutions in industry and society" (ibid) to tackle global challenges.
- Economic impact: Seeks to support all types of innovation, including breakthrough advancements, and to enhance the market adoption of innovative solutions.

The upcoming EU Framework Programme for Research is currently referred to as "FP10" as a placeholder until an official name is decided. Although "FP10" is still several years away, the ongoing interim evaluation of Horizon Europe serves as a foundation for beginning discussions on the future direction of European research, technology, and innovation policies beyond 2027. It is likely that the evaluation of impact from engaged research will build on the foundation laid down in Horizon Europe.

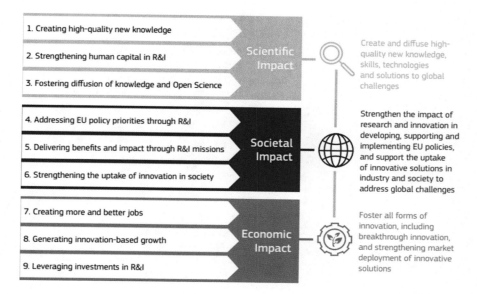

Fig. 4.6 Tracking performance along key impact pathways towards impact. The Horizon Europe monitoring and evaluation framework objectives translate into three complementary impact categories (scientific, societal, and economic), which reflect the non-linear nature of research and innovation investments. (Reprinted from European Commission 2018b)

As discussed in Chap. 2, the KEF provides an excellent framework for helping providers of higher education in England to better understand and improve their own performance in engaged research. The third iteration of the KEF, called KEF3, was published in June 2023, and it provides an updated set of metrics which along with narrative statements will be used to monitor knowledge exchange activities (Table 4.2).

4.3 Overcoming Silo Thinking

All stakeholders of an engaged research ecosystem, both within and outside academia, must overcome tunnel vision and embrace a holistic approach to solving complex problems in the twenty-first century. This requires that silo thinking is replaced with adaptive, holistic systems thinking. Researchers and public and private partners in society must overcome sole reliance on discipline-specific research and engage more widely with colleagues from other disciplines and partners in the public. Engaged research in the future can overcome academic mono-disciplinary silo thinking and become agile and interdisciplinary through several transformative approaches.

Funders may increase incentives for interdisciplinary and intersectoral work further through grant mechanisms that stipulate that researchers step outside

Table 4.2 Summary of the perspectives and metrics that will be used in KEF3

KEF3 perspective title	KEF3 metric description
Research partnerships	Contribution to collaborative research (cash) as proportion of public funding
	Co-authorship with non-academic partners as a proportion of total outputs—amended to include trade journals. Data provided by Elsevier
Working with business	Innovate UK income (KTP and grant) as proportion of research income
	[a]HE-BCI contract research income with non-SME business normalised by HEP income
	HE-BCI contract research income with SME business normalised by HEP income
	HE-BCI consultancy and facilities income with non-SME business normalised by HEP income
	HE-BCI consultancy and facilities income with SME business normalised by HEP income
Working with the public and third sector	HE-BCI contract research income with the public and third sector normalised by HEP income
	HE-BCI consultancy and facilities income with the public and third sector normalised by HEP income
Continuing professional development (CPD) and graduate start-ups	HE-BCI CPD/CE income normalised by HEP income
	HE-BCI graduate start-ups rate by student FTE
Local growth and regeneration	HE-BCI regeneration and development income from all sources normalised by HEP income
	Additional narrative/contextual information—updated for KEF3 March 2023
IP and commercialisation	HE-BCI estimated current turnover of all active firms per spin-out surviving at least 3 years
	HE-BCI average external investment per spin-out surviving at least 3 years
	HE-BCI licensing and other IP income as proportion of research income
Public and community engagement	Self-assessment-based metric—score updated for KEF3 in March 2023 (optional)
	Additional narrative/contextual information—updated for KEF3 March 2023

(Adapted from Research England 2023) (Contains public sector information licensed under the Open Government Licence v3.0. http://www.nationalarchives.gov.uk/doc/open-government-licence/version/3/)
[a]Higher Education Business and Community Interaction (HE-BCI) survey collects financial and output data related to knowledge exchange each academic year and has been running since 1999

disciplinary silos and work with public, industry, and non-governmental partners. The European Union has a long tradition of challenging researchers to look beyond national and disciplinary boundaries to form their research teams.

In higher education institutions, interdisciplinary research centres already drive this research forward. In the future, even greater emphasis will be placed on inviting external stakeholders into research partnerships. This may alter power relationships and generate new forms and mechanisms of co-production.

Still, many universities lack strong visions for new interdisciplinary and inter-professional education programmes that foster agile learning and produce graduates not constrained by professional or disciplinary boundaries. There is a reluctance to promote this type of twenty-first-century "renaissance scholarship" to address the complexities of our time. New cross-disciplinary and modular programmes and degrees, flexible academic structures and processes, mixed discipline faculty appointments, and new career development and evaluation metrics may change this.

Globalised research networks (e.g. UNA Europa; Universitas) may also generate new capacity-building offerings and research partnerships.

Perhaps, the most vital element for a departure from silo thinking is a mindset change, a cultural shift at scale. Collaboration across disciplines and engagement with societal stakeholders must be understood as essential to solving complex global problems (e.g. climate change, one health pandemics, human-machine interaction). This shift will involve recognising the value of diverse perspectives and breaking down the traditional hierarchies that privilege some disciplines. Engaged research, co-production, and interdisciplinarity require capacity building in relevant collaboration and communication skills. This includes fostering the ability to work effectively with people from different backgrounds, understanding the culture, language, experiences, values, expectations, and methodologies of other disciplines and stakeholders, and developing shared goals.

Engaged research of the future will have to be increasingly focused on solving complex, real-world problems requiring modular and integrated research designs. Research questions will be framed around societal challenges (e.g. sustainable development, one health) rather than discipline-specific theories and approaches. This also means stronger partnerships with industry, government, and community organisations are needed to bundle resources and expertise while retaining academic freedom.

Open science and open-access publishing are at the forefront of democratising research. Open science strives to make research findings and data freely available to everyone. Cross-disciplinary open data-sharing platforms involving large datasets from multiple topics will facilitate new cross-disciplinary collaborations and provide avenues for artificial intelligence in complex data analyses. Many datasets are already available to researchers anonymously and held by transnational or national statistics offices.

The future of engaged research is contingent upon foresight and strategic leadership. University administrators, policymakers, and funding agencies must collaborate to formulate policies that foster interdisciplinary research. These entities will synchronise their strategies to facilitate the formation of multidisciplinary teams, endorse open access, and prioritise funding for research addressing societal challenges. Leadership is pivotal in cultivating a culture of collaboration, incentivising interdisciplinary projects, and ensuring the requisite infrastructure is established.

At the international level, governments and organisations such as the United Nations and the World Health Organization could spearhead global research initiatives necessitating interdisciplinary collaboration, thereby contributing to a cohesive global research ecosystem. University leaders, including presidents and deans, will be instrumental in nurturing a multidisciplinary culture by implementing policies encouraging collaboration, instituting awards and recognition for interdisciplinary work, and promoting diversity in research methodologies.

Engaged research can transcend academic silo thinking and become more agile, responsive, and interdisciplinary, but this shift necessitates dedicated efforts from institutions, researchers, and policymakers. The benefits will be substantial, equipping academia and non-academic partners to tackle the complex challenges of the future with greater efficacy. The outlined strategies can potentially establish a novel ecosystem of engaged research characterised by enhanced collaboration, innovation, and responsiveness to real-world issues.

4.4 Refining Research Practices

As engaged research practices expand, a growing need exists to refine, standardise, and enhance sharing of successful processes underpinning these activities. There needs to be more than theory shared. The practical, on-the-ground processes and their developments need greater exchange and sharing. Implementation is typically a learning curve. Resources are wasted when these learnings are instead considered failures and not shared in the community for a variety of reasons. "Best practices" cannot be determined without the sharing of practices. In this section we share learnings and suggestions from our own experiences.

4.4.1 Achieving Equality, Diversity, and Inclusion

One of the frontiers for engaged research in higher education is to foster a culture that acknowledges the need to reflect diverse voices and perspectives equitably and inclusively. Universities are committed to equality, diversity, and inclusion (EDI). Achieving EDI in engaged research requires alignment with EDI-supportive policies, building partnerships with external stakeholders advocating for minority and marginalised populations, and ensuring that HEIs have diverse leadership in research management. All research-relevant policies should be "EDI-proofed".

In concrete terms, this means whether funding and career opportunities reflect diversity, the infrastructure is usable and accessible to all and appropriate to work with external partners on a long-term basis. The policies should enable co-production in research between academic and external partners over time, requiring adequate recognition of the collaborative nature of the work by research ethics, finance, and human resources departments. Diverse perspectives should also be visible in the administrative and academic leadership and allow the career progression of research managers and educational scholars from diverse backgrounds supported through mentorship and seed funding for participatory and engaged research initiatives. Research education should include methodological approaches in participatory research with stakeholders from underrepresented communities, foster experiential learning, and provide a rich set of practical EDI engaged research case studies. Partnership with external community partners also requires the incorporation of cultural competency training. Universities should also consider offering research funding for projects that engage diverse communities and address issues related to equity and inclusion. This includes providing grants specifically for participatory research that fosters diversity of perspectives. Universities, as key generators of new knowledge, are also responsible for disseminating knowledge broadly and equitably to stakeholders through accessible and inclusive processes. This includes providing open access to research publications, producing community-friendly reports, and using multiple languages, formats, methods, and media to communicate findings. Partners representing underserved communities should be invited routinely to co-organise dissemination and public-facing engagement events, co-present and co-author academic and non-academic outputs, and be seen to lead discussions on the value and impact of research visibly.

Universities should involve community partners in the dissemination process, allowing them to co-present findings, co-author reports, and lead discussions on research implications. This ensures that diverse perspectives are not only included in the research process but also the sharing of knowledge. Universities must also be seen as influential voices in achieving system change through engagement with policymakers, funders, and the more comprehensive public and private partners to promote diversity in research. Academics play a critical role in organising lectures and conferences on the value of EDI. They can lead by example and ensure that students are taught by community representatives and other stakeholders, and are involved in co-production activities even at undergraduate level (Molosi-France and Dipholo 2022). By leveraging their institutional influence, universities can push for systemic changes, encouraging inclusive research practices across the academic sector. Finally, universities can develop metrics to assess the impact of their engaged research initiatives on diversity and inclusion. Regular evaluation and feedback loops can help universities identify areas for improvement, ensure that their efforts to foster diversity are practical, and make them publicly accountable.

4.4.2   Maintaining Openness and Dynamism in Engaged Research

Besides considering diversity from an EDI perspective, engaged research also requires constant vigilance and openness toward new and fresh perspectives from different stakeholders. Participatory research, at times, needs to distinguish between advocacy and research. Advocacy has a particular function and may or may not rely on research evidence to pursue the goals of its cause. Engaged research should not be mistaken for advocacy, even though it may have shared goals and intended impacts on communities. Advocates can be powerful voices for communities and stakeholders. However, the sole reliance on the same advocates is not representative of the diversity of constituents. Therefore, engaged research needs to pause and reflect on who is and is not part of the research processes and whose voices and perspectives are heard or not heard. Universities and academics must be open to changes in co-production relationships, regularly refresh advisory committees, and open up capacity-building and research opportunities to new individual and organisational partners. This is necessary to maintain vigour, innovation, and equity in their partnerships.

4.4.3   Ethical Engagement Practices

The ethical implications of engaged research are complex and multifaceted. Researchers must navigate issues related to power dynamics, informed consent, and the potential for unintended consequences. To address these challenges, institutions, civil society organisations, and professional bodies should develop and disseminate best practices for ethical engagement. This includes tools for directly addressing potential ethical and research integrity risks, creating tools for assessing the ethical implications of research projects, and establishing mechanisms for ongoing ethical oversight. There is a gap in the knowledge base on the ethical considerations of engaged research. It is often assumed to be "morally correct" to engage members of the public in research. However, there are potential risks that need to be acknowledged, considered, and minimised. A part of research ethics is to consider the potential risks and well-being of research teams including public or community-based collaborators. Whereas RPOs may have policies, procedures, and resources to mitigate many of these risks for staff or student researchers, members of the public involved in research (who are not classified as staff) may not be covered by these policies. It is therefore important to consider how to address, mitigate, and minimise potential risks to public contributors (see Dorris and MacLoughlin 2024 for a more detailed discussion).

4.5   Capacity Building Within and Beyond HEIs

The long-term success of engaged research will depend on the development of supportive policy for all stakeholders. To ensure the sustainability of engaged research, there must be a concerted effort to build capacity among all stakeholders involved. This includes not only RPOs but also societal partners, policymakers, and the broader public.

4.5.1 Training and Professional Development

Researchers need access to training that equips them with the skills and knowledge necessary for effective engagement. This includes training in communication, facilitation, project management, and ethical considerations. Furthermore, the units responsible for research enhancing practices need to be informed about the practices core to engaged research. Researchers can help research ethics committees (RECs) or Institutional Review Boards (IRBs) to fully assess proposals by giving them the necessary information to do so. It is important for researchers to clearly explain the rationale, approach, and how they have considered and mitigated all risks, including potential risks arising via engaged research, when applying for ethical review. Not every REC will have expertise in engaged research or be as familiar with the intricacies of involving external stakeholders as the applicants themselves. The ability to communicate the rationale, values, principles, and potential risks of engaged research is important not just for research dissemination but also for building up networks of partners. Professional development opportunities to upskill should be available at all career stages, from early-career researchers to senior academics.

There has been much discussion regarding training opportunities for publics and community stakeholders. A core value of engaged research is the different perspectives brought from different stakeholders. There are typically two diverse views on the training of community partners. The first advocates for upskilling public stakeholders to a level where they can confidently engage with academic researchers on the academic's (or other professional's) level. This involves high-level training in nomenclature, key theories, and current state of the art in the research area. This requires intense dedication and commitment on behalf of the public stakeholder. These stakeholders are often called "lived experience experts" indicating that in addition to lived experience they also have the technical knowledge of the area of research. In converse, there are those that advocate for little training on the side of the public or community stakeholders, unless specifically requested by said stakeholders. This camp focuses on the need for the research culture to change. Research professionals and RPOs are responsible for being able to engage at the level "where people are". The responsibility is to skill the researchers rather than the community. The onus is on the researchers and RPOs to be flexible to the community rather than trying to fit the community into the traditional academic or corporate research structures.

4.5.2 Empowering Societal Partners

Engaged research is a two-way street, and societal partners must also be empowered to contribute effectively. This is not meant in a patronising way, rather it refers to tangible efforts to address structural and systemic power imbalances and disadvantages. It may involve creating opportunities for capacity building within community organisations, and ensuring that partners have access to the resources they need to participate fully. However, the responsibility for this is not solely on the RPO. Charities and CBOs are autonomous organisations and have their own goals, values, and principles. The relationships between CBOs and research institutions must be of benefit to both organisations, and there must be buy-in from both sides. If the upskilling, support, and resourcing comes solely from the RPO it may not adequately reflect the needs of CBOs.

The third sector must direct their own development in this space to forward their own agenda. Conversely, the third sector is generally under-resourced, and engagement with RPOs to improve research may not be high on their priorities. This has resulted in the emergence of organisations that are addressing this gap. That is, organisations in the third sector who recognise the potential benefits of engaged research and are taking up the mantle of providing support in order to create a more equitable environment. One example of these organisations is European Patients' Academy on Therapeutic Innovation (EUPATI) and their national platforms, which provide education and training to increase the capacity and capability of patients and patient representatives to understand and meaningfully contribute to medicines research and development (Pushparajah et al. 2016).

Governments and research funding bodies should develop policies that explicitly recognise and support engaged research and the inclusion of non-traditional research actors. This may include incorporating engagement criteria into funding calls, creating incentives to prioritise engagement activities, and developing policies that protect the autonomy and rights of societal partners. This is advancing, with some funding calls widening eligibility to societal partners, and including their eligibility equal to that of RPOs and industry partners. This should help to build capacity in charities and CBOs and assist in equalising power dynamics amongst multi-sector research partners.

4.6 Interplay of Public Engagement and Engaged Research

Building a culture of engaged research requires ongoing public engagement and education. This can be achieved through outreach activities, public lectures, and the inclusion of engagement topics in educational curricula (Ní Shúilleabháin et al. 2021). By fostering a broader understanding of the value of engaged research, we can help to build public support and ensure that engagement becomes a normalised and expected aspect of the research process.

We consider public engagement in research as encompassing a wide spectrum of activities. It has evolved over time with an increasing focus on a two-way process with the goal of generating mutual benefit for the research institution and the public and civic organisations they engage. Outreach, public consultation, and public education of science are important foundations that can build to engaged research, even though they in and of themselves are not engaged research. A key test of engaged

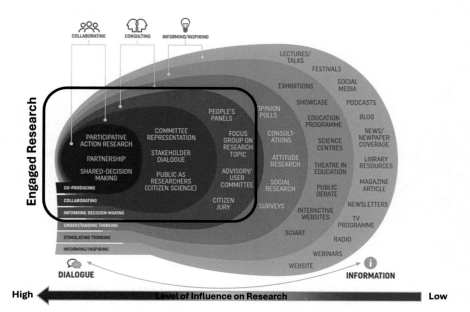

Fig. 4.7 UCD "Avocado" of public engagement activities adapted to highlight engaged research and how different activities have different levels of influence on research. The Avocado was based on Wellcome Trust's public engagement onion (The Wellcome Trust "onion" model is © the Wellcome Trust and is licensed under Creative Commons Attribution 2.0 UK. https://creativecommons.org/licenses/by/2.0/uk/)

research within the wider framework of public engagement is the influence on the decision-making processes of research. Activities, initiatives, and collaborations that include two-way, mutually benefit interactions that influence research typically fall within engaged research (Fig. 4.7). These activities focus on two-way knowledge exchange. Outreach and educational activities on the other hand are typically primary one-way knowledge exchange, from researchers to the public, and consultations are one way knowledge exchange from the public to researchers. The scope for informing what knowledge is exchanged is one sided, whereas engaged research by its very nature always has two-way knowledge exchange.

Outreach activities, however, serve as crucial conduits for bridging the divide between research and society. Engaging with the public through outreach activities enhances the accessibility of research insights and can lead to fostering a reciprocal exchange of ideas. For researchers, this platform offers an opportunity to refine their communication skills, broaden their societal interactions, and receive insight about how the public perceive their research. For the public, access to expert knowledge helps critical thinking skills, and engagement with contemporary issues.

Outreach activities are also important for another, commonly overlooked, reason: shared spaces. Researcher-research or research-industry collaborations often arise out of interactions in shared spaces such as conferences or professional events. These events play a fundamental role in fostering successful collaboration by providing environments conducive to the exchange of ideas, interdisciplinary engagement, and the development of synergistic relationships (de Leon and McQuillin 2020). They act as hubs for interaction, allowing individuals from different backgrounds with shared interest to engage in informal dialogue and structured problem-solving (Su et al. 2016). Often, non-professionals are excluded from conferences and professional events. This results in their exclusion from spontaneous knowledge sharing, which is often critical for addressing complex challenges that require multifaceted approaches. In some disciplines, conferences are opening up to interested publics and communities, most commonly in health research, when the patient involvement movement is relatively more supported and advanced. However, this is not standard practice across all disciplines. Thus, outreach activities can play a role in bringing professionals and non-professionals with shared interests together. Done well, they can create environments that help cultivate a sense of community and trust among professionals and non-professionals, which is fundamental for the progression of these relationships to collaborations. Ultimately, outreach can serve as a vital mechanism for strengthening the connection between research and society.

4.7   The Future Ecosystem of Engaged Research

Undoubtedly, engaged research is here to stay and will likely expand over the coming decades. We will see engaged research mature in that policies and procedures will be increasingly shared, adopted, evaluated, and modified. The exact nature of engaged research in the future is difficult to predict.

Macro-political developments will influence the future of engaged research. Engaged research is predicated on cooperation, democratic decision-making, and the proactive inclusion of minorities (Guerrini et al. 2018). Engaged research can only thrive within a democratic framework that supports collaboration. It may not thrive everywhere. As described in Chap. 1, engaged research relies on different historical traditions, and we may see other forms of engaged research evolve worldwide.

Despite numerous methodological examples, there remains ambiguity about whether engaged research will be more than ethos or tokenistic practice and can lead to transformation at scale. It often appears more as an aspiration than a fulfilment, with processes seeming engaged but outcomes not necessarily reflecting mutual benefits on a significant scale. Structural and power imbalances may persist, preventing true transformation, and conservatism and fear of change may form a backlash. Engaged research posits to improve research quality, and a large body of descriptive and anecdotal evidence suggests that this may be true as costly mistakes can be avoided in the research process. While important, the sole focus on outcomes may overlook the process's intrinsic value. There is a risk of manualisation of engaged research through "toolboxes" and "quick fixes", which counter the need for genuine commitment, reflective practice, and open dialogue among research partners.

The desire for standardisation might lead to oversimplification or deter more involvement in the research process due to perceived complexity. Only some public stakeholders may be invited to join research teams. Over-reliance on established relationships can hinder fresh perspectives that ad hoc relationships might bring to dialogues between academic and public stakeholders. Typically, these would be easy to reach and communicate with, well-educated and relatively low maintenance. Avoiding professionalisation is essential to ensure inclusivity in the research process. At the institutional level, universities with greater appreciation of the value of engaged research may be more willing to adopt policies and procedures for stakeholder engagement. Caution is warranted to ensure that policies and procedures remain agile and flexible enough to meet the needs of new and changing partnership constellations.

New stakeholders will enter the research space in the future, and new engagement processes will evolve. It will be essential to maintain openness in engaged research for changes in how partners will plan, conduct, and disseminate or implement research findings. New technologies will accelerate the process. Artificial intelligence will play a significant role in connecting stakeholders across the globe, facilitating engagement processes, and speeding up tailor-made knowledge outputs. Human and machine actors will work together in new and unprecedented ways. There is substantial potential to work with local and global publics more efficiently. Real-time translation will allow for engagement with non-English-speaking communities. The development of groundbreaking assistive technologies will likely enable engagement with stakeholders who have been systematically excluded from research and decision-making processes because of cognitive or communicative impairments, research literacy or linguistic barriers, and researchers' unwillingness to look for assistive tools.

Technology will also transform research administration, from HR via research ethics to research communication and dissemination (Liu et al. 2023). Artificial intelligence can connect researchers and teams in new ways and quickly identify expertise. We should, however, be vigilant and cautious so that stakeholder voices, experiences, and agencies do not get lost in the increasing reliance on artificial intelligence and technologies. There needs to be a continuous reflection on who may not be visible or is not included in the research process.

In this book we have attempted to characterise the status of engaged research and the different ways how changes in policy, higher education, and civil society have begun to transform research. Specifically, the book has provided some illustration of how university policies and procedures are beginning to change to facilitate open, engaged, inclusive, and innovative science.

References

Canada, Government of. Canadian Net-Zero Emissions Accountability Act SC 2021, c 22. 2021.

Citizen Initiative on Climate, Association of the Citizens' Climate Report. Recommendations for German climate policy. 2021.

Clark C, Cluver M, Fishman T, Kunkel D. 2024 Higher education trends. Deloitte center for government insights [Internet]. 2024. Available from: https://www2.deloitte.com/us/en/insights/industry/public-sector/latest-trends-in-higher-education.html.

Commission D-GfRaIE. Responsible research and innovation: Europe's ability to respond to societal challenges. 2012 2012-10-04.

Commission Recommendation (EU) 2023/499 of 1 March 2023 on a Code of Practice on the management of intellectual assets for knowledge valorisation in the European Research Area. 2023.

de Leon FLL, McQuillin B. The role of conferences on the pathway to academic impact: evidence from a natural experiment. J Hum Resour. 2020;55(1):164–93.

Dorris E, MacLoughlin D. Research ethics committees and public and patient involvement. In: Minogue V, Salsberg J, editors. Meaningful and safe: the ethics and ethical implications of patient and public involvement in health and medical research. Ethics Press; 2024.

Elstub S, Farrell D, Carrick J, Mockler P. Evaluation of Climate Assembly UK. Newcastle upon Tyne. 2021.

European Commission DGRI. Reforming research assessment: the agreement is now final. In: Innovation D-GfRa. Brussels: European Commission; 2022a.

European Commission DGRI. European Research Area policy agenda—Overview of actions for the period 2022–2024: Publications Office of the European Union. 2022b.

European Commission T. A new ERA for research and innovation. Brussels: European Commission; 2020.

European Commission: DGRI. OSPP-REC—Open Science Policy Platform Recommendations: Publications Office. 2018a.

European Commission: DGRI. A new horizon for Europe—impact assessment of the 9th EU framework programme for research and innovation. Publications Office; 2018b.

European Commission: DGRI. Commission staff working document. Impact assessment accompanying the document proposals for a regulation of the European Parliament and of the council establishing Horizon Europe—the framework programme for research and innovation, laying down its rules for participation and dissemination. Publications Office. 2018c.

European Commission: DGRI Valorisation policies—Making research results work for society—Intellectual property fosters innovation and societal impact: Publications Office. 2021.

European Commission: DGRI. Valorisation policies—Code of practice on citizen engagement—Commission recommendation: Publications Office of the European Union. 2024.

European Commission: DGRI, Pottaki I, Monaco F, Articolo R, Martinez E, et al. Fostering knowledge valorisation through citizen engagement. Publications Office of the European Union; 2024.

European Commission: Directorate-General for E. Level(s) and the new European Bauhaus: Publications Office of the European Union. 2022.

European Commission: Directorate-General for Employment SA, Inclusion, Stott L, Jakubowska K, Pavlovaite I, Chowdhury N, et al. The ESF and community-led local development—lessons for the future—ESF transnational cooperation platform community of practice on social innovation. Publications Office of the European Union; 2022.

Fiorino DJ. Citizen participation and environmental risk: a survey of institutional mechanisms. Sci Technol Hum Values. 1990;15(2):226–43.

Gibbons M, NCSES. Universities report largest growth in federally funded R&D expenditures since FY 2011. NSF [Internet]. 2022;23(303) Available from: https://ncses.nsf.gov/pubs/nsf23303

Guerrini CJ, Majumder MA, Lewellyn MJ, McGuire AL. Citizen science, public policy. Science. 2018;361(6398):134.

Ireland Government of National Dialogue on Climate Action (NDCA). In: Department of the Environment, editor. Dublin 2021.

Ireland Government of Climate Conversations 2024. In: Department of the Environment. Dublin. 2024.

Jah YC. Stakeholder-engaged research: a multidisciplinary historical analysis. Research for All. 2024;8(1)

Liu BL, Morales D, Roser-Chinchilla J, Sabzalieva E, Valentini A, Vieira do Nascimento D, et al. Harnessing the era of artificial intelligence in higher education: a primer for higher education stakeholders. UNESCO; 2023.

MacDonogh H, Davies C, Smith K. Rethinking policy impact. 2022.

MITECO. Asamblea Ciudadana para el Clima: Una España más segura y justa ante el cambio climático š Cómo lo hacemos?: Technical report. 2022.

Molosi-France K, Dipholo K. Community based participatory research: a ladder of opportunity for engaged scholarship in higher education. Journal of Contemporary Issues in Education. 2022;17(2):111–22.

Ní Shúilleabháin A, McAuliffe F, Ní SÉ. 'Bottoms up': a case study on integrating public engagement within a university culture. Research for All. 2021;5(2)

NIH N. NIMHD Community-Based Participatory Research Program (CBPR). 2024. Available from: https://grants.nih.gov/grants/guide/rfa-files/rfa-md-15-010.html

Owen R, Macnaghten P, Stilgoe J. Responsible research and innovation: from science in society to science for society, with society. In: Emerging technologies: ethics, law and governance; 2012.

Pedersen DB, Krieger K. An evaluation framework for institutional capacity of science-for-policy ecosystems in EU Member States. Developing an evaluation framework for science-for-policy ecosystems 2023;

Pushparajah DS, Geissler J, Westergaard N. EUPATI: collaboration between patients, academia and industry to champion the informed patient in the research and development of medicines. Journal of Medicines Development Sciences. 2016;1(1)

Reed MS. The research impact handbook. 2nd ed. Huntly, Aberdeenshire: Fast Track Impact; 2018.

Research England. Knowledge exchange framework decisions for the third iteration. 2023. Available from: https://www.ukri.org/publications/knowledge-exchange-framework-kef-decisions-for-the-third-iteration/

Shelley-Egan C, Gjefsen MD, Nydal R. Consolidating RRI and Open Science: understanding the potential for transformative change. Life Sciences, Society and Policy. 2020;16(1):7.

Song H, Markowitz DM, Taylor SH. Trusting on the shoulders of open giants? Open science increases trust in science for the public and academics. J Commun. 2022;72(4):497–510.

Stirling A. Risk, uncertainty and precaution: some instrumental implications from the social sciences. Negotiating environmental change. 2003:33–76.

Su X, Wang W, Yu S, Zhang C, Bekele TM, Xia F. Can academic conferences promote research collaboration? Proceedings of the 16th ACM/IEEE-CS on joint conference on digital libraries. Newark, New Jersey, USA: Association for Computing Machinery; 2016. p. 231–2.

Transforming Our World: The 2030 Agenda for Sustainable Development., ST(02)/T77. 2015.

UIS, UNESCO Institute for Statistics, 'Research and development expenditure (% of GDP)', UIS. Stat Bulk Data Download Service. 2024. <apiportal.uis.unesco.org/bdds>.

UKRI. UKRI's equality, diversity and inclusion strategy .2023. Available from: https://www.ukri.org/publications/ukris-equality-diversity-and-inclusion-strategy/

USA, House Committee on Oversight and Government Reform, 'Crowdsourcing and Citizen Science Act 15 U.S.C. § 3724'. 2016.

USA DoHHS. CDC prevention research Centres 2021. Available from: https://www.cdc.gov/prc/index.htm

White House T. Open government policy collection. Obama White House Archives [Internet]. 2009–2014. 2024. Available from: https://obamawhitehouse.archives.gov/open/about/policy

Appendix: Method for Identifying Engaged Research Publications

The below query was built in Elsevier Scopus to analyse the volume of academic publications relating to engaged research.

Date of search: 21 Aug 2024
Scopus Search Terms:

> TITLE-ABS-KEY ("engaged research" OR "engaged scholarship" OR "community engaged research" OR "community and stakeholder engagement" OR "Community-Based Research" OR "Participatory Research" OR "Community-engaged research" OR "Community engagement" OR "Patient and public involvement" OR "adolescent carer" OR "citizen science" OR "Patient engagement" OR "community engagement" OR "stakeholder engagement" OR "citizen involvement" OR "Public Participation Network" OR "Person and public involvement" OR "Patient involvement" OR "Deliberative democracy" OR "end user engagement" OR "Community-engaged research" OR "citizen assembly" OR "patient participation" OR "Public and patient involvement (PPI)" OR "Public and patient involvement") AND PUBYEAR > 2013 AND PUBYEAR < 2024

Index